Preface

"Much ado about nothing"?

The human immunodeficiency virus (HIV-1) began to spread among the homosexual population in the USA in the late 1970s and it was not until 1981 that physicians in New York and at CDC Atlanta recognized the new clinical syndrome AIDS (acquired immune deficiency syndrome), alerting the world to a new and fatal infection. Only with the isolation of a causative virus in 1983 did it become apparent that, as with other infective agents, routes of transmission could be envisaged. During the early 1980s the Shakespearian preface title may have summarized widespread opinion of AIDS, at least in most countries outside the USA. But it is quite apparent now that infection with HIV represents one of the greatest health problems of our time. The World Health Organization estimate that 10 million people worldwide are infected with HIV. Research into all facets of HIV is proceeding at a dramatic pace and this volume is produced to relay current strategies for prevention and therapy of AIDS and AIDS-related infections.

Specific diagnostic tests for HIV infection, e.g. detection of viral antigens and anti-core antibodies, have been developed and the use of these tests may indicate which patients should be treated with anti-retroviral therapy, perhaps even before full-blown AIDS develops. Within two years of the isolation of HIV a nucleoside analogue zidovudine (formerly known as azidothymidine) had been identified and shown to inhibit the virus in the laboratory and to slow the remorseless clinical deterioration of AIDS patients. New, potent and selective inhibitors of HIV replication such as sulphated polysaccharides and dideoxynucleosides offer promise for the future. In contrast, HIV presents serious theoretical problems to vaccine development and no effective vaccine has yet been found.

Patients with AIDS develop life-threatening opportunistic infections, including pneumocystis pneumonia, toxoplasmosis, bowel infections with numerous pathogens, and cytomegalovirus (CMV), fungal and mycobacterial infections. Current diagnostic procedures and available therapies for these infections are also discussed in this volume. In pneumocystis pneumonia, cotrimoxazole and pentamidine are reasonably effective, but because of high rates of side effects in AIDS patients new agents are needed. In CMV infections, gancyclovir and foscarnet are promising antiviral agents, especially for the treatment of retinitis.

There is room for cautious optimism about the development of effective therapies for AIDS and AIDS-related infections. In the absence of effective vaccines antiviral chemotherapy will be pivotal in controlling the AIDS epidemic.

ADRIAN BINT
JOHN OXFORD
Stratford-on-Avon, UK
April 1988

Contents

Journal of Antimicrobial Chemotherapy (1989) **23**, *Suppl. A*, 1–7

The biology and epidemiology of HIV infections

Jonathan Weber

Department of Medicine, Royal Post-graduate Medical School, Hammersmith Hospital, Ducane Road, London W12 0HS, UK

The world now has a pandemic of infection by the human immunodeficiency virus type I (HIV-1). More recently, a focus of epidemic HIV-2 infection in West Africa has been noted and this too is spreading internationally. HIV-2 closely resembles a simian lentivirus, SIV; SIV isolates have now been made from African (but not Asian) old world monkeys and SIV infection in macaques may provide the best animal model for HIV. All of these viruses share a tropism for the CD4 molecule, which is intimately involved in their pathogenesis. The immune response to these viruses has yet to demonstrate any protective immunity.

Introduction

It is difficult to exaggerate the significance of the HIV epidemic which has swept through the world in seven years. The World Health Organization (WHO) now estimate that over 5 million people are already infected by HIV, and portrays a grim picture of continued spread of this virus. Cases of AIDS have now been reported from over 140 countries, out of 160 in WHO, and countries without AIDS are now rare. While the USA leads with the largest number of reported AIDS cases, over 50,000, central and eastern Africa is thought to have a greater covert problem. South America is poised to be hit hard by HIV, and Brazil already reports the second highest AIDS toll, after the USA. If transmission of HIV were to stop today, new cases of AIDS would still be a growing problem into the middle of the next decade. In the absence of a vaccine or cure, AIDS will change the practice of medicine in this country, and in all others. The only sources of optimism lie in the WHO Global Programme on AIDS (the GPA), and in the immense investment in AIDS research internationally.

The AIDS viruses

The human immunodeficiency virus type 1 (HIV-1) was first reported by Françoise Barré-Sinoussi and her colleagues in Luc Montagnier's laboratory at the Institut Pasteur in May 1983 (Barré-Sinoussi *et al.*, 1983). Subsequently, research in Gallo's laboratory in Washington in 1984 demonstrated that this virus was unequivocally the cause of AIDS and related conditions (Cheinsong-Popov *et al.*, 1984; Gallo *et al.*, 1984; Popovic *et al.*, 1984). The HIV viruses are retroviruses, RNA viruses replicating through a DNA proviral intermediate, generated by a virally encoded RNA-directed DNA polymerase (reverse transcriptase). Retroviruses are common infections of

1

animals, infecting vertebrates as evolutionary diverse as primates and reptiles (see review, Wong-Staal & Gallo, 1985).

Classification of retroviruses

Retroviruses are classified by their morphology on electron microscopy, and by their clinical manifestations, into three categories. Spumaviruses (foamy viruses) have been isolated from man and primates, and cause a characteristic foamy vacuolation of cells in culture; they have not yet been associated with any specific disease. The second group, the oncoviruses, are associated with tumour development in a wide range of animals, and there is one human example, HTLV-1, the human T-cell leukaemia/lymphoma virus. The third group, the lentiviruses, are associated with disease of prolonged latency between infection and overt clinical manifestation. The first member of this group, the visna/maedi virus of sheep, causes pneumonia and neurological disease; goats may be infected by the caprine arthritis/encephalitis virus, and horses by the equine infectious anaemia virus. HIV belongs to this group and all these viruses are associated with lifelong persistent infection. More recently, it has been recognized that primates are infected with a range of lentiviruses of the simian immunodeficiency virus (SIV) group (Hunsman & Schneider, 1988), and newly discovered lentiviruses infect cattle (BIV), and cats (FIV) (Pedersen et al., 1987).

HIV-1 is now pandemic. HIV-2, a related but distinct virus recognized since 1985 in West Africa, appears to be more closely related to the SIV group, and is relatively localized to this area at present. HIV-2 was first demonstrated serologically in Dakar, Senegal, by Kanki and others in 1985, and first isolated by Clavel in 1986 (Kanki et al., 1985; Clavel et al., 1986). HIV-2 has now been reported from at least seven west African countries, including Senegal, Gambia, Ivory Coast, Guinea-Bissau, Cape Verde Islands and Mali (Kanki et al., 1987). It has also been found sporadically in the UK, in many European countries and in the USA. Given the capacity of HIV-1 to travel, it is inevitable that HIV-2 infection will become more widespread over time, and new assays are currently being developed for the sero-diagnosis of HIV-2 infection. As discussed below, there is some evidence that the natural history of HIV-2 infection may differ in detail from HIV-1, although both viruses lead to an indistinguishable clinical syndrome, AIDS.

Animal models

HIV-1 infects humans, and leads to persistent infection in chimpanzees after experimental inoculation, as yet without overt disease (but see below). HIV-2, by contrast, will also infect macaques and baboons, but probably only in a transient manner. As there is no evidence of AIDS developing after animal inoculation with HIV, the favoured animal model for AIDS will be the SIV infection in macaques. SIV has been isolated from macaques, mangabeys, mandrills and African green monkeys, mostly in primate colonies (Hunsman & Schneider, 1988). The SIV macaque isolate (SIV$_{mac}$) causes an AIDS-like syndrome (Simian AIDS, SAIDS) on inoculation into healthy macaques, with a latency of 10–14 months. These viruses have been identified in wild, caught, Old World monkeys, and the close similarity of SIV to HIV-2 suggests that a zoonosis is the likeliest origin of the HIV epidemic. However, the human and

Table I. Genomic relationship between HIV-1, HIV-2 and SIV$_{mac}$

	HIV-1bru	HIV-2rod	HIV-leli	HIV-lmal
HIV-1$_{bru}$	—	59·4	94·4	92·0
HIV-2$_{rod}$	59·4	—	61·6	59·0
SIV$_{mac}$	59·0	83·6	58·2	59·2

Numbers refer to the % genome similarity.

simian viruses are sufficiently different to point to a long evolutionary diversity. Table I shows that the SIV isolate is more closely related to HIV-2 than HIV-1.

Pathogenesis

The pathogenesis of disease following HIV infection may be broken down into primary and secondary effects (Table II).

The most consistent feature of HIV infection is a gradual diminution of CD4+ T-lymphocytes from the peripheral blood, both quantitatively and qualitatively. As the majority of CD4+ cells are T-helper lymphocytes, the major action of HIV is to paralyse the cellular immune system, which requires the T-helper cell for the initiation of cytotoxic T-cell killing of virally infected cells or cancerous cells. The loss of the T-helper lymphocytes, because of HIV infection, leads to loss of cellular immune surveillance and hence the appearance of virally induced tumours from unopposed clonal expansion of virally transformed cells. Additionally, cellular immune depletion leads to loss of control of endogenous viral, fungal and protozoal infections, which may proliferate and present as an 'opportunist' infection. The other side of the cellular immune equation, the antigen-presenting cell (e.g. monocyte, macrophage) may also be HIV-infected, and functionally abnormal. It is still unclear what further role the infected macrophage plays in HIV pathogenesis, but the specific nature of the infections in AIDS implies that local immune phenomena, such as failure of surveillance in the lung, specifically predisposes to Pneumocystis carinii pneumonia. The T-helper lymphocyte also plays a role in B-cell help, and in initiating new B-cell responses to soluble antigen. HIV-infected subjects are hypergammaglobulinaemic, and this represents a polyclonal activation of existing B-cell populations; the ability to make new useful antibodies is greatly impaired by HIV infection.

In addition, it is possible to categorize the cellular response to HIV infection into:

Table II. Pathogenesis of disease following HIV infection

Primary effects
    Quantitative and qualitative decrease in infected cells
    Impaired cellular immunity
    Impaired immune surveillance
    Direct pathology in the CNS, gut and elsewhere

Secondary effects
    Opportunist infections
    Virally mediated tumours

(a) cell tropism; (b) effect of HIV genome expression on cell: (c) immune response to infected cells, and (d) host factors e.g. genetic susceptibility.

Viral life cycle

The HIV virus enters susceptible cells by binding to a specific receptor on the cell surface, the CD4 antigen. After entry into the cytoplasm, the virus uncoats, and the viral reverse transcriptase generates a DNA provirus, which may then enter the cell nucleus, and through the action of viral integrases, the viral DNA integrates into the host cell chromosomes at a random site. The replication of the virus requires an integrated genome, and hence infection by HIV is persistent and likely to be lifelong. Viral replication leads to the formation of eight principal viral proteins, which assemble at the cell surface, and leave the cell by budding. All of these surface proteins are immunogenic in the course of natural infection. The proteins of HIV comprise the structural components, the core (p24) and the envelope (gp41); the enzymes, and the regulatory genes which act as positive and negative controllers of viral replication.

The identification in 1984 of the CD4 molecule as a major component of the cellular receptor, by Klatzman and Dalgleish has proved an important hallmark in HIV research (Dalgleish *et al.*, 1984; Klatzmann *et al.*, 1984). Subsequently in 1986, Maddon and others showed that transfection of the CD4 gene alone conferred susceptibility to HIV infection in cells which do not constitutively express CD4 (Maddon *et al.*, 1986). The definition of the HIV receptor allows the tissue distribution of HIV to be accurately defined.

Cells infectable by HIV

The effect of HIV on cells *in vitro* ranges from cell death through lysis, cell fusion or senescence to continuous viral production without any cytopathicity. Clearly, there are cellular factors which influence the outcome of HIV infection at a cellular level, and several studies have demonstrated that the amount of CD4 on the cell surface is critically related to the HIV cytopathic effect (Table III). In addition, the role of the HIV regulatory genes, particularly the *tat*, *art* and *3'orf* genes appear to play a central role in the repression and stimulation of HIV viral replication. The *3'orf* gene seems to play a critical role in the down-regulation of viral replication, and the expression of this gene may partly explain the long latency between infection and disease. It is now

Table III. CD4 levels obtainable on cell surfaces

Cell type	CD4 positive (%)	HIV susceptibility	Distribution
T-helper lymphocyte	100	+++	blood, lymph node
B-lymphocyte	5	+	blood, lymph node
Monocyte	10	++	blood, lymph node
Macrophage	10	++	lung, gut, brain
Glial	mRNA+[a]	±	brain
Colon	mRNA+[a]	±	gut

[a]Not detectable by immunofluorescence on cell surface but mRNA positive.

clear that all of the lentiviruses contain equivalent genes to the HIV regulatory genes, and a better understanding of the molecular basis of HIV pathogenesis is rapidly being developed.

The time course of HIV infection

Prospective studies of HIV infection in groups of homosexual men, intravenous drug abusers and transfusion-related HIV infection have yielded broadly comparable results in terms of the probability of AIDS developing. At six years of follow-up in the San Francisco homosexual cohort, 35% of HIV-infected subjects went from an asymptomatic state to develop AIDS (Moss *et al.*, 1987). At this time point, there is a 7% per annum probability of AIDS developing. There is no sign that the cumulative total of AIDS is levelling out, and much speculation exists as to the ultimate proportion of HIV-infected subjects who will go on to develop HIV-related disease. While the medical establishment is divided into pessimists and optimists, with some forecasting 100% mortality from HIV infection, the prognosis can only be determined by prospective studies. While this is frustrating to doctors and patients alike, the central question of the prognosis of HIV infection will have to wait until the end of the century, or longer. As discussed later, the emergence of effective antiviral drugs may result in modification of HIV infection in early stages. If drugs such as zidovudine (formerly azidothymidine, AZT) are widely used in HIV infection, the true natural history of HIV may never be known. Only in a unique disease such as AIDS can this bizarre situation occur, where modification of a disease's unknown natural history is attempted.

After infection with HIV, there is a 'window' period where infection is latent, and there is no detectable immune response to the virus. This period may last 4–12 weeks and in rare cases may be very much longer. This is followed by a detectable presence of HIV p24 antigen in the peripheral blood for a short period, often one to two weeks, immediately before the emergence of the humoral immune response. The first antibody response to core (p24) proteins and to envelope proteins (gp41) are more or less simultaneous. The envelope response continues throughout the duration of HIV infection, rising to a maximum titre after six to nine months of infection, and maintained thereafter. The core response to the virus declines in association with the emergence of symptomatic disease (Weber *et al.*, 1987).

The natural history of HIV-2 infection is even less clear than for HIV-1, for as yet there are no longitudinal studies. It is clear that HIV-2 leads to AIDS, as a number of AIDS patients in West Africa have had no other infection. Some workers have stressed that HIV-2 appears less pathogenic in cell culture, and that the great majority of HIV-2 infected subjects are totally asymptomatic (Clavel, 1987). However, at any one time, the majority of HIV-1 patients are also well, and a study of HIV-1 infection in New York in 1981 would have suggested that the virus was relatively non-pathogenic. Cohort studies have now been established in West Africa and preliminary answers to the relative pathogenicity of the two viruses will be available from 1990.

Prognostic factors in HIV infection

Faced with a lengthy period between infection and the development of overt disease, and the maintenance of a proportion of long-term healthy survivors, the factors associated with progression of HIV disease are of considerable importance. Now that antiviral therapy is developing, the identification of those asymptomatic patients at most risk to AIDS is of great importance. In addition, HIV-infected subjects require the best prognostic information available.

Early prognostic markers are centred on the CD4+ lymphocyte, as all AIDS cases are associated with depletion of CD4+ cells to low levels. The serial measurement of CD4+ cells in HIV infected subjects shows a gradual diminution over time in those progressing to AIDS. Other studies have suggested that all asymptomatic subjects show a loss of CD4+ lymphocytes over time. This leads to the uncomfortable notion that all subjects have markers of progression. However, there is a wide variation in the CD4 count in asymptomatic, infected subjects, and serial assessment is required rather than the absolute total at any one time. This is particularly true in sexually acquired HIV infection, where the time point of infection is not generally known. Indirect markers of cellular immunity, such as delayed type hypersensitivity (DTH) to recall antigens are abnormally reduced in HIV infection, but several studies have shown that homosexual men may have anergic DTH responses in the absence of HIV. Other indirect markers such as β-2 microglobulin levels (a component of the class I Major Histocompatibility Complex, MHC, molecule, and a ligand for cytotoxic T-cells) are increased in HIV infection, and thus higher levels predict for more rapid evolution to AIDS. These markers are easier to use in retrospect, as the range can be wide. Several studies have in addition used cross-sectional groups of patients in different clinical stages of HIV infection. This is misleading as prognostic factors can only be accurately assessed on longitudinal cohorts of subjects followed over time, as they progress through the stages of AIDS.

It is now possible to titre the humoral response to both core and envelope proteins of HIV separately and an assay for viral antigenaemia now exists. The time course of infection shows that the anti-envelope antibodies are conserved, but the anti-core antibodies decline before the development of disease-between CDC group III and group IV. Subsequent to this, anti-core (anti p24) antibodies decline and there is detectable p24 core antigen in the serum. Monitoring the viral antigen and anti-core antibodies represents the first virally specific prognostic markers, and these are becoming widely used.

References

Barré-Sinoussi, F., Chermann, J. C., Rey, F., Nugeyre, M. T., Chamaret, S., Gruest, J. *et al.* (1983). Isolation of a T-lymphotropic retrovirus for a patient at risk for acquired immune deficiency syndrome (AIDS). *Science* **220**, 868–70.

Cheinsong-Popov, R., Weiss, R. A., Dalgleish, A., Tedder, R. S., Shanson, D. C., Jeffries, D. J. *et al.* (1984). Prevalence of antibody to human T-lymphotropic virus type III in AIDS and AIDS-risk patients in Britain. *Lancet ii,* 477–80.

Clavel, F. (1987). HIV-2. *AIDS* **1,** 156–62.

Clavel, F., Guétard, D., Brun-Vézinet, F., Chamaret, S., Rey, M.-A., Santo-Ferreira, M. O. *et al.* (1986). Isolation of a new human retrovirus for West African patients with AIDS. *Science* **233**, 343–6.

Dalgleish, A. G., Beverley, P. C. L., Clapham, P. R., Crawford, D. M., Greaves, M. F. & Weiss, R. A. (1984). The CD4 (T4) antigen is an essential component of the receptor for the AIDS retrovirus. *Nature* **312**, 763–7.

Gallo, R. C., Salahuddin, S. Z., Popovic, M., Shearer, G. M., Kaplan, M., Palker, T. J. *et al.* (1984). Frequent detection and isolation of cytopathic retroviruses (HTLV-III) from patients with AIDS and at risk of AIDS. *Science* **224**, 500–3.

Hunsman, G. & Schneider, J. (1988). The primate lentiviruses. *AIDS* **2**, 1–15.

Kanki, P. J., M'Boup, S., Ricard, D., Barin, F., Denis, F., Boyce, C. *et al.* (1987). HTLV-IV and HIV in West Africa. *Science* **236**, 827–31.

Kanki, P. J., McLane, M. F., King, N. W., Letvin, N. L., Hunt, R. D., Sehgal, P. *et al.* (1985). Serological identification and characterisation of a macaque T-lymphotropic retrovirus closely related to HTLV-III. *Science* **228**, 1199–201.

Klatzmann, D., Champagne, E., Chamaret, S., Gruest, J., Guétard, D., Hercend, T. *et al.* (1984). T-lymphocyte T4 molecule behaves as the receptor for human retrovirus LAV. *Nature* **312**, 767–8.

Maddon, P. J., Dalgleish, A. G., Clapham, P., McDougal, S., Weiss, R. A. & Axel, R. (1986). The T4 gene encodes the AIDS virus receptor and is expressed in the immune system and the brain. *Cell* **47**, 333–48.

Moss, A. R., Osmond, D., Baccheti, P., Chermann, J. C., Barré-Sinoussi, F. & Carlson, J. (1987). Risk factors for AIDS and HIV seropositivity in homosexual men. *American Journal of Epidemiology* **125**, 1035–47.

Pedersen, N. C., Ho, E. W., Brown, M. L. & Yamamoto, J. K. (1987). Isolation of a T-lymphotropic virus from domestic cats with an immunodeficiency syndrome. *Science* **235**, 790–5.

Popovic, M., Sarngadharan, M. G., Read, E. & Gallo, R. C. (1984). Detection, isolation and continuous production of cytopathic retroviruses (HTLV-III) from patients with AIDS and pre-AIDS. *Science* **224**, 497–500.

Weber, J. N., Clapham, P. R., Weiss, R. A., Parker, D., Roberts, C., Duncan, J. *et al.* (1987). Human immunodeficiency virus infection in two cohorts of homosexual men: neutralising sera and association of anti-*gag* antibodies with prognosis. *Lancet* **i**, 119–22.

Wong-Staal, F. & Gallo, R. C. (1985). Human T-lymphotropic retrovirus. *Nature* **317**, 395–403.

Journal of Antimicrobial Chemotherapy (1989) **23**, *Suppl. A*, 9–27

Potential target sites for antiviral inhibitors of human immunodeficiency virus (HIV)

J. S. Oxford, A. R. M. Coates, D. Y. Sia, K. Brown and S. Asad

Department of Medical Microbiology, The London Hospital Medical College, Turner Street, London E1 2AD, UK

The rapid identification of anti-HIV compounds in the laboratory following the isolation of the causative virus in 1983 and their subsequent use in the clinic was not unexpected. Three decades of previous work had established a scientific basis for the evaluation of antiviral compounds. However, no antiviral yet discovered can cause total blockade of a virus replicating in a cell. The combination of properties of HIV including latency, antigenic and biochemical variation is unusual and the virus represents a daunting challenge for chemotherapy. But at least 90 antiviral compounds have been discovered, many inhibiting the virus reverse transcriptase. Other targets for inhibition are possible including viral regulatory gene products, viral protease and endonuclease enzymes but compounds for initial study will have to be found by random searching. X-ray crystallography of HIV proteins will shortly be possible, enabling the commencement of a more molecular specific search for inhibitors. Meanwhile, advantage can be taken of comparative nucleotide sequences of the HIV-1 and -2 genomes to test short oligonucleotides as potential inhibitors of mRNA transcription. The *pol* gene also has a zinc finger amino acid sequence suggesting that chelation chemotherapy may have a potential role. In the absence of HIV vaccines, and associated theoretical problems in their development, antiviral chemotherapy is expected to occupy a central role in combating the AIDS epidemic.

Introduction

The rapid identification and deployment of a number of inhibitors of HIV-1 virus replication (Figure 1), particularly nucleoside analogues (McCormick *et al.*, 1984; de Clercq *et al.*, 1986; Mitsuya & Broder, 1986, 1987; Lin, Schinazi & Prusoff, 1987; Mitsuya *et al.*, 1987) is a striking example of the practical potential of antiviral chemotherapy. Thus within two or three years of the discovery of HIV-1 as the causative agent of AIDS (Barré-Sinoussi *et al.*, 1983), several inhibitors of the essential reverse transcriptase (RT) enzyme of the virus had been used in the clinic (reviewed by Yarchoan *et al.*, 1986; Fisch *et al.*, 1987; Yarchoan & Broder, 1987) to treat patients with AIDS. Most of these compounds had been investigated previously as anti-viral compounds in the laboratory against other retroviruses (reviewed by Hirsch, 1988), but certainly the potential and selectivity *in vitro* of at least one of these molecules, namely zidovudine (azidothymidine; AZT), although it was first synthesized in 1964, had not been fully realized until recently. An HIV gene map, and the potential targets for antiviral activity are shown in Table I. The science and practice of antiviral chemotherapy have been difficult (reviewed by Bauer, 1985) but the efforts of

9

Inhibitors of HIV RT enzyme

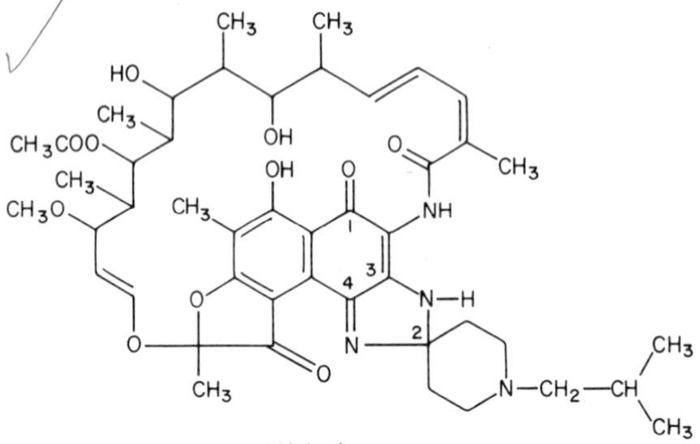

Rifabutin

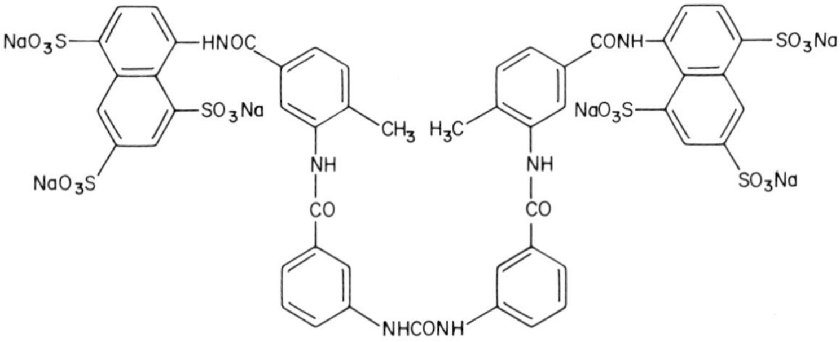

Suramin

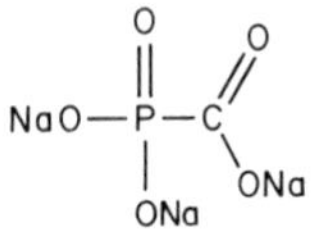

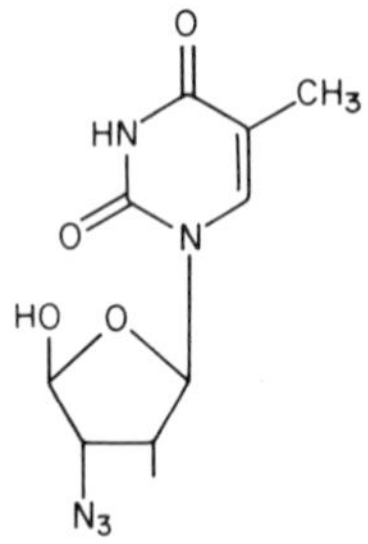

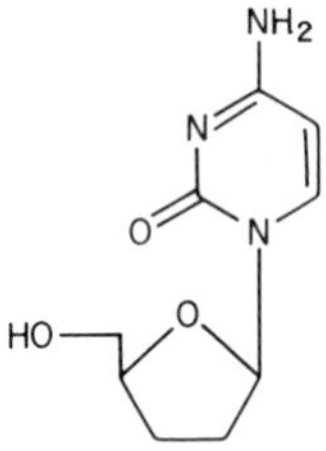

Foscarnet

Zidovudine

Dideoxycytidine

Inhibitors of viral protein processing

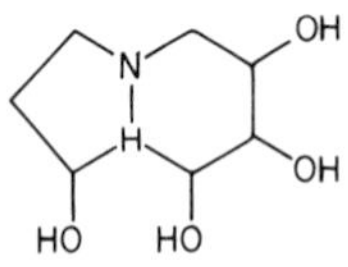

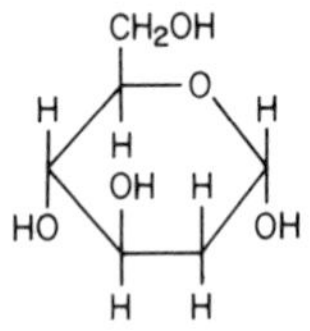

Castanospermine

2-Deoxy-D-glucose

Compounds acting at an unknown stage of viral replication

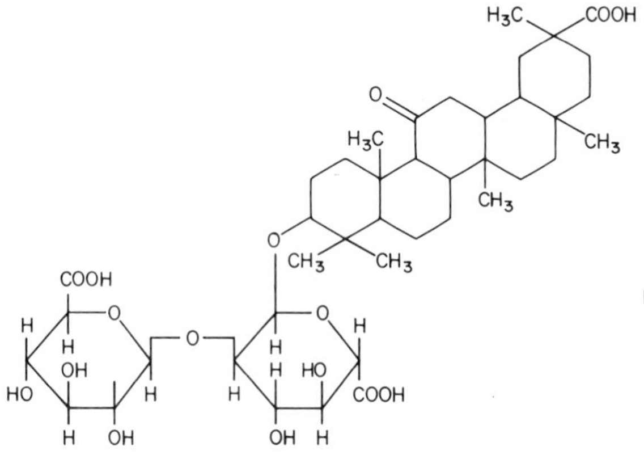

Glycyrrhizic acid

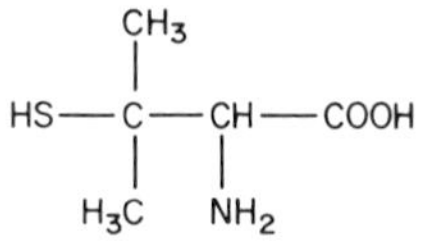

D-Penicillamine

Direct effect on virions

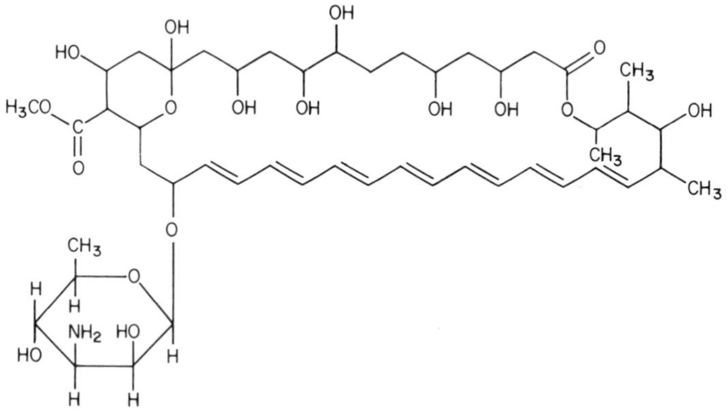

Amphotericin B methyl ester

Inhibitors of early events of virus infection of cells

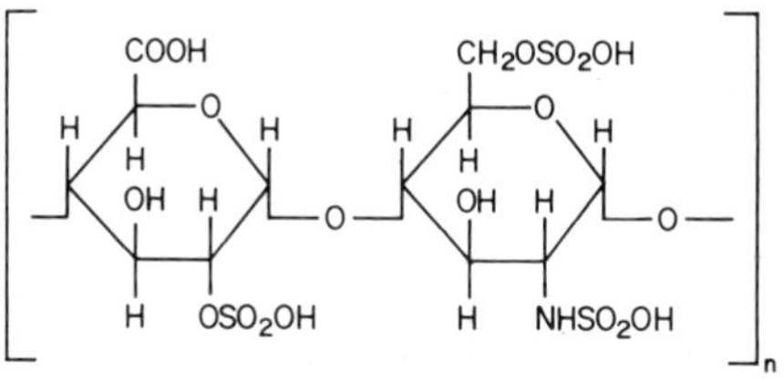

Heparin

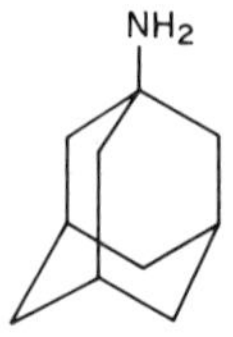

Amantadine

Figure 1. (a) Inhibitors of HIV replication and cell infection.

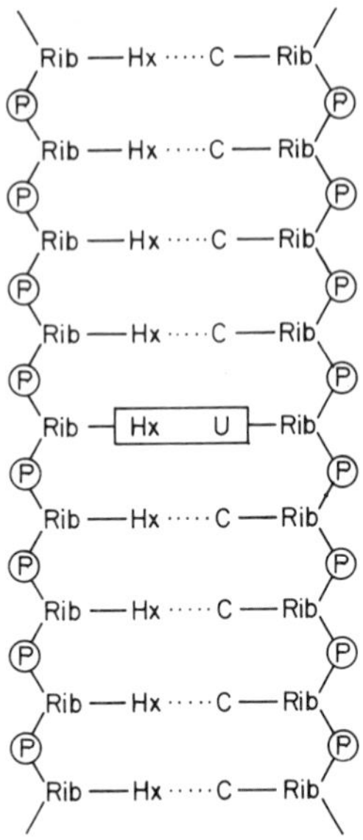

Figure 1. (b) Inhibition of viral RNA transcription or mRNA translation. Mismatched $(I)_n.(C_{12}.U)$ Ampligen: the poly (inosinic acid $[(I)_n]$ strand is composed of hypoxanthine (Hx), ribose (Rib) and phosphate ⓟ) whereas the poly(cytidylic acid) strand contains at an average 1 uracil (U) per 12 cytosine (C) bases $[(C_{12}.U_n]$. U in its keto configuration cannot form a base pair with Hx. Modified from de Clercq, 1987.

many contributors over the past four decades have laid the foundations with well developed in-vitro procedures, animal models and, in the final analysis, use of placebo controlled clinical trials.

In contrast, attempts to develop vaccines against HIV-1 have not been successful to date (reviewed by Minor, 1988, this Volume, p. 55). Indeed there are indications both theoretical and practical from studies of other animal lentiviruses that this approach, normally so successful in the development of vaccines (reviewed by Oxford & Oberg, 1985), may not be effective for lentiviruses in general and HIV in particular.

In the context of antiviral therapy, one of the most significant biological properties of the HIV-1 virus is its ability to integrate a DNA copy of its diploid RNA genome into the chromosome of the host cell. This means that once a single cell in a person has been infected with the AIDS lentivirus, the viral genetic information will be carried *ad infinitum*. Unfortunately, relatively few of the infected cells are actually killed by HIV-1 and hence cells continue to release fresh virus and infect further cells. Some susceptible cells have a short half-life of days or weeks but others such as dendritic macrophages may persist for decades. Probably many cells in circulation are infected although only 1 in 10,000 is actually activated at any one time to produce virus. When or whether clinical AIDS eventually develops is a matter not clearly understood, although available data would suggest that over a ten year period 60–70% of such infected persons will develop the clinical syndrome. The major challenge facing chemotherapists therefore is either to eradicate the integrated HIV-1 genome from all infected cells in the body or to suppress the later transcription of the genetic information of the integrated proviral DNA. In this case an antiviral may have to be

Table I. HIV genes as potential targets for antivirals

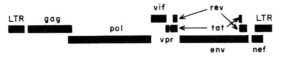

Genes	Function	Potential as target for antiviral
tat	Transactivator of viral proteins	Excellent
rev	Regulates expression of virion proteins	Excellent
vif	Determines virus infectivity	Excellent
vpr	Unknown	?
nef	Reduces virus expression.	No
gag	Core or capsid proteins	?
pol	Protease, reverse transcriptase and endonuclease (integrase)	Excellent e.g. zidovudine ddc foscarnet
env	Envelope glycoprotein – virus attachment and fusion events	Good.
LTR	Long terminal repeat	?

used prophylactically for a lifetime and hence would have to be non-toxic. Such an immense undertaking of a complete cure of an infected individual is just conceivable with antiviral chemotherapy, but not, most would concede at the present, with a vaccine strategy. The other property required of an anti-AIDS drug is to inhibit the wide range of HIV-1 and HIV-2 viruses which are circulating in some communities. This antiviral spectrum could, with benefit, also include HTLV-1 virus which is also spreading, albeit more slowly.

Can the lessons of comparative virology help towards the development of HIV chemotherapy?

Many important questions relevant to antiviral chemotherapy remain unanswered. Are individuals infected with a mixture of genetic variants of HIV, and is this the case for other RNA virus infections? Could a single individual harbour HIV with a range of susceptibilities to antiviral compounds? Another important question is whether the virus can undergo many replicating cycles in the absence of integration into the host cell chromosome. Antiviral chemotherapists already have experience of viruses which incorporate latency in the life cycle; herpes virus, and an even more epidemic virus than HIV, influenza A. For neither of these has an anti-viral been discovered which will totally inhibit virus replication, either *in vitro* or in human infections. Unlike the situation in anti-bacterial chemotherapy, a few virus particles always appear to be able

Table II. Points of action of antiviral inhibitors of HIV-1

Life cycle of virus	Known or potential compounds
Free virions	Disinfectants (Spire *et al.*, 1984), AL-721 (Sarin *et al.*, 1985) polymannoacetate (McDaniel & McAnalley, 1987). Potentially interesting point of action and amenable to ELISA for screening
Adsorbing virions	Pentapeptides[a] (Pert *et al.*, 1986). Di or tripeptides could block receptor binding site on gp120. Soluble CD4 protein with N terminus KKVVLGKKGD inhibits virus replication (Hussey *et al.*, 1988). Dextran sulphate (de Clercq, 1988, this volume).
Penetration and uncoating	Silicotungstate may modify cell membrane (Jasmin *et al.*, 1973). Lysosomotropic agents such as ammonium chloride and amantadine inhibit HIV replication but may act additionally at budding stage (qv). Virus probably enters cell by 'fusion from without'. Permeability changes in infected cells (Pasternak, 1987) may allow selective entry of antivirals into virus infected cells.
Reverse transcriptase (RT) enzyme of virus	A favourite and successful target. AZT[a] dideoxy cytidine[a], Foscarnet[a], rifabutin[a] (Anand *et al.*, 1986), Suramin[a] (Mitsuya *et al.*, 1984), HPA 23[a] (Rozenbaum *et al.*, 1985). Studies are well advanced to define functional areas of the molecule and to use X-ray crystallography to help design new inhibitors
Circularization of viral DNA: viral integrase	No known inhibitors but integrase enzyme is a particularly interesting target. Viral integrase has a typical 'zinc finger' structure of a zinc metalloenzyme and hence thiosemicarbazone and related chelators may inhibit (Oxford & Perrin, 1974, 1977). D-penicillamine[a] has antiviral effect (Sarin, 1987) 1987). Tat protein binds zinc (Frankel *et al.*, 1988).
Virus induced protease	Important function in processing virus structural and nonstructural polypeptides. Inhibited by pepstatin A (Katch *et al.*, 1987) and an important target.
Viral regulatory gene products *tat, rev* *vif, vpr*	No known inhibitors. No specific biochemical test yet available for screening

Table II—*continued*

Life cycle of virus	Known or potential compounds
Transcription of pro-viral DNA	Synthetic 'antisense' oligonucleotides with sequences complementary to proviral DNA may inhibit transcription to mRNA or virion RNA translation Ribavirin[a] may inhibit mRNA primary and elongation.
Intracellular processing of viral glycoproteins	An alkaloid from *Castanospermium australe* inhibits glucosidase processing of viral gp120
Virion budding	Amantadine and related molecules. Interferons[a] may act at this stage (Ho *et al.*, 1985). Morphological changes at the post budding stage may form an additional target. (see Fig. 1)

[a]Clinical trials completed or in progress.

to replicate in the presence of the highest concentrations of anti-viral. These 'breakthrough' virus particles are not necessarily 'drug resistant'.

In the short term, what are the prospects for developing a range of new antivirals against HIV-1? HIV-1 has many of the structural and biological characteristics of viruses which in the past have proved very amenable to chemotherapy, such as the herpes group (Bauer, 1985). In general, viruses with a relatively large genome and with a complex biological life cycle involving subtle control elements during replication have proved to be more easily inhibited than viruses with a less complex life cycle such as the small RNA picornaviruses. Furthermore, the intense research interest in lentiviruses will mean that every type of scientific approach used against other viruses over the last three decades of antiviral chemotherapy will be re-examined in the context of this new epidemic virus. Therefore, it would be surprising if a tremendous diversity of inhibitors is not discovered and found to inhibit the virus directly or to inhibit the development of AIDS indirectly by restoring immune function.

This brief review summarizes the action of antivirals known to inhibit other viruses at varying stages of the life cycle and where possible, emphasizes points relevant to anti-HIV-1 drug development. Some sections of the review will be speculative. This exercise in comparative virology, with potential anti-AIDS drugs fitted into a wider perspective of antivirals, may stimulate new investigations into classes of inhibitors which are already well known to antiviral chemotherapists but not necessarily to AIDS specialists. The preceding paper in this Volume (Weber, 1988, this Volume p. 1) has reviewed the various stages in the life cycle of HIV in some detail and therefore will not be repeated here.

Antiviral molecules binding to free virions

Inhibitors which bind to free virus particles have been little investigated in the past, with the notable exception of rhinoviruses, where a number of quite potent molecules bind to the external proteins of the virus (Smith *et al.*, 1986) and effect virion stability, often increasing it, and hence inhibit later stages of virus uncoating. Potential anti-AIDS drugs which act as inhibitors of this kind would be detected by screening with modern ELISA binding techniques. Possibly the only compound known at present, apart from disinfectants (Schuster, Cohn & McKeeking, 1986) which could affect virus stability is AL-721, a mixture of neutral glycerides, phosphatidylcholine and phosphadidylethanolamine which is thought to reduce the cholesterol content of viral membranes, causing changes in membrane fluidity which interfere with virus attachment (Sarin *et al.*, 1985).

Inhibition of virus attachment to susceptible cells and subsequent virus entry and uncoating

In the last five years X-ray crystallography has delineated the three dimensional configuration of amino acids in and around receptor sites on external glycoproteins of influenza and other viruses (Wilson *et al.*, 1981; Smith *et al.*, 1986). These receptor-site host cell interactions are known to be very specific and, of course, a vital first step for virus attachment. The first antiviral study at the molecular level of an inhibitor binding in a receptor binding area has been published (Smith *et al.*, 1986), providing new impetus for the design of antiviral inhibitors binding to virions. Work in progress includes the study of potential inhibitors of influenza neuraminidase, where X-ray crystallography data of the viral protein and the enzyme active site have already been published (Colman *et al.*, 1987). The potential for designed anti-AIDS drugs is considerable. Already, short peptides have been shown to inhibit HIV-1 virus attachment to cells (Pert *et al.*, 1986). Pert *et al.* (1986) investigated the HIV inhibitory effects of a pentapeptide of the terminal amino acids of the viral gp120 envelope glycoprotein. Virus attachment is thought to occur through this pentapeptide sequence, which is similar for all HIV isolates. More recently Hussey *et al.* (1988) have described inhibition of HIV replication and syncytium formation by a soluble CD4 polypeptide expressed in a baculovirus system with the N terminal sequence KKVVLGKKGD. Apart from the logical approaches of synthesizing short peptides to compete with the viral sequence involved in binding it is possible that other molecules, found by random screening, may be equally effective inhibitors. In the long term, study of the interactions of the viral receptor site on gp120 and the cell CD4 receptor respectively by X-ray crystallography should enable logical construction of inhibitors of the correct shape, size and charge. At this stage even the screening of a complete series of di or tripeptides using plastic pin—ELISA technology may give useful new leads (Geyson *et al.*, 1987). Inhibitors of this kind would be of the maximum size to fit into the influenza HA receptor binding pocket (Wilson *et al.*, 1981).

  Short peptides as antivirals are a relatively modern area of interest to antiviral chemotherapists although in an early study, carried out before the linear sequence of amino acids was known, a series of short peptides were shown to inhibit replication of measles and influenza viruses *in vitro* (Choppin, Richardson & Scheid, 1983). Most interestingly, with influenza virus HA, sequence specific peptides were subsequently synthesized. Like HIV gp120, influenza HA is a fusion protein but catalyses fusion of viral and host cell membranes in intracellular vacuoles at low pH. Hexapeptides of the fusion sequence at the N terminus of HA2 inhibited influenza viral replication *in vitro* but not *in vivo*. One of the major problems with this approach is to prevent degradation of the peptide *in vivo* and this was not overcome in the case of the influenza study. A synthetic octapeptide of sequence TGAVVNDL corresponding to the carboxy terminus of the small subunit of herpes ribonucleotide reductase inhibits enzyme function but, indicative of the problems to be confronted with HIV, failed to inhibit herpes virus replication *in vitro* (Dutia *et al.*, 1986).

There is some controversy concerning the precise way HIV enters a cell after attachment to the CD4 receptor. Earlier data suggested a viropexis mechanism, followed by a low pH endosomal vacuole stage (Maddon *et al.*, 1986), in a scheme rather similar to influenza (reviewed by Stuart-Harris, Schild & Oxford, 1985). In this case virus uncoating would be inhibited by lysosomotropic agents such as amantadine. However, other data suggest a pH independent 'fusion from without' mechanism, akin to paramyxoviruses which can proceed at physiological pH (Stein *et al.*, 1987; McClure, Marsh & Weiss, 1988). Amantadine and related ammonium ions do inhibit HIV replication *in vitro*, but perhaps at a later stage of the virus cycle. Even the precise point of action of amantadine against influenza is not completely established after three decades of work and, as an additional complication, the compound may exert its effects at more than one place in the virus life cycle (see below). Finally, it is quite possible that certain laboratory strains of HIV differ in their cell entry mechanisms, with the susceptible cell under test being an additional variable. The laboratory experience with influenza has shown that experiments to demonstrate the virus entry mechanism are equivocal in interpretation. Even if virus particles are observed by electron microscopy to be entering in one way, it would still be possible for other particles to actually infect the cell by an alternative pathway.

HIV gene transcription and genome integration

A unique and yet essential feature of the life cycle of the AIDS lentivirus is the reverse transcription by a viral enzyme of the RNA genome into a DNA copy. This viral DNA is circularized and integrated into host chromosomal DNA (the so-called provirus DNA). At later stages the proviral DNA is activated (Nabel *et al.*, 1988) and transcribed into viral mRNAs which code for viral structural proteins. RNA to be incorporated into new virus particles also has to be faithfully transcribed from the proviral DNA. Thus, several viral coded enzymes are essential for viral replication and there is a general consensus that they could form vulnerable targets for inhibitors. How the first inhibitory compound of the integrase is to be discovered is unknown, although it is quite likely that random screening, which is being carried out now at the rate of many thousands of compounds each week worldwide, will provide the first lead.

Viral coded reverse transcriptase

Already, the virion associated reverse transcriptase (RT) has been highlighted as a target. The RT gene has been cloned (Larder *et al.*, 1987) and the gene product can be produced in large quantities. Several molecules of very diverse molecular structure such as zidovudine (reviewed by Hirsch, 1988), foscarnet, (Oberg, 1986), suramin, rifabutin (Anand *et al.*, 1986) and HPA 23 (Dormont *et al.*, 1985) have been shown to cause inhibition of the enzyme *in vitro*. To date only one of these inhibitors, the nucleoside analogue zidovudine, has shown clear antiviral activity in the clinic in placebo controlled trials, although clinical trials are now in progress with a related compound, dideoxycytidine (Yarchoan *et al.*, 1988).

A whole family of 2',3' dideoxynucleosides exists and it is apparent that they may vary considerably in their antiviral and anti-cellular activities. Removal of the oxygen at the 3' carbon of the sugar of 2' deoxyadenosine changes the molecule into a powerful antiviral compound, 2',3' dideoxyadenosine. But a further change at the 5' carbon (2',3' and 5' trideoxyadenosine) abrogates the antiviral activity. Since cytidine, thymidine, guanosine and adenine can all be modified, the search for the compound with the most balanced combination of properties (antiviral versus toxic) may be a long one. But already some interesting molecules in this grouping of nucleoside analogues have been tested in the laboratory including a series of 2',3' didehydro 2'3' dideoxyribonucleosides (Balzarini *et al.*, 1987), and 3' deoxythymidin-2' ene (Lin *et al.*, 1987). To give further perspective, zidovudine was chosen initially as a lead compound on in-vitro antiviral action, yet subsequent clinical studies have shown how difficult it may be to separate antiviral effects from anticellular toxicity. In the cell zidovudine can reduce 2' deoxycytidine triphosphate levels and this pyrimidine starvation may be a cause of the observed bone marrow suppression noted in AIDS patients treated with the compound (Richman *et al.*, 1987). These compounds require a host cell TK enzyme to phosphorylate them to the triphosphate which is the molecule that actually inhibits viral reverse transcriptase activity by virtue of DNA chain blocking. One positive aspect of this necessity for host cell enzymes to activate the compounds is that lentiviruses cannot revert to drug resistance by a mutation in a viral TK gene as can herpes viruses (Coen, Chiou & Gibbs, 1986).

Inhibition of viral mRNA function

Relatively short oligonucleotides with a length of 12 nucleotides have been shown to inhibit HIV replication in cell culture (Zamecnik *et al.*, 1986; Matsukura *et al.*, 1987). Similar molecules have also been shown to inhibit another retrovirus, Rous sarcoma virus (Zamecnik & Stephenson, 1977). The oligonucleotides can be synthesized with a base sequence complementary to conserved regions of the HIV provirus DNA. In theory they would be expected to hybridize with active or transcribing viral DNA whereas they would not hybridize with DNA in a normal cell unless, by chance, a nucleotide sequence common to a retrovirus was present. Such hybridization of an 'anti-sense' molecule would block transcription and hence inhibit the production of viral mRNA (Melton, 1985) and viral proteins. Alternatively, it is conceivable that these 'anti-sense' molecules could also inhibit translation directly from viral mRNA. Obviously with such a large HIV genome of around 10,000 nucleotides, considerable judgement will be required to choose a suitable sequence for targeting, whilst additional problems are cellular entry of the molecules, the possibility that even after entry they may be preferentially sequestered in the cytoplasm rather than the nucleus where they need to be to hybridize to proviral DNA and, finally destruction by cellular enzymes. Favourite areas along the HIV genome for 'anti-sense' oligonucleotide attack would be at the start codons of the *gag*, *env* or *pol* genes or at the splice donor acceptor and primer binding regions. A particularly interesting approach would be the targeting of a toxic molecule either attached to the specific oligonucleotide (Eiklid, Olsnes & Pihl, 1980), or activated by it after specific binding (Uhr, 1984; Toulmé *et al.*, 1986; Thuong *et al.*, 1987; Uhlenbeck, 1987). We are initiating in-vitro studies using

Table III. Antisense oligonucleotides with potential anti HIV activity

---

vif gene (4574–4591)

T AGT AAT CCCT AAT ACCT	Antisense
AT CAT T AGGGAT T AT GGA	HIV-1 lav
. . . . . C . . A . . C	HIV-1 rod
. . T . . C . AA	SIV mac

nef gene (8348–8361)

AT AT T CT ACCCACC	Antisense
T AT AAGAT GGGT GG	HIV-1 lav
. GC . . T	HIV-2 rod
. . C . . T	SIV mac

RNA primer binding site

ACCGCGGGCT T GT CCCT G	Antisense
T GGCGCCCGAACAGGGAC	HIV-1 lav
. . . . T	HIV 2
. . . .	SIV mac

RNA primer binding site and 3′ extension

CT T GT CCCT GAACT T T CGCT	Antisense
GAACAGGGACT T GAAAGCGA	HIV-1 lav
. . . . GAA . .	HIV-2
. . . . G . A . .	SIV mac

Oligonucleotides are synthesized with a base sequence complementary to conserved regions of HIV-I, HIV-2 and SIV DNA. They may be protected from intracellular degradation by addition of side groups.

'anti-sense' oligonucleotides (Oxford, J. S. & Coates, A., unpublished data) corresponding to areas of the genome of HIV-1 which are also shared by HIV-2 and SIV, thus enabling animal model studies to be performed of any active molecules in the monkey. Nuclease resistant analogues of oligo deoxynucleotides have been synthesized whilst additionally some oligonucleotides with non-complementary sequences also inhibit HIV *in vitro*, particularly a 28 unit phosphorothioate oligodeoxycytidine. Synergistic activity was shown with a 14 unit molecule with a non complementary sequence to HIV and 2′,3′ dideoxyadenosine (Matsukura *et al.*, 1987).

Inhibition of low molecular weight polypeptide gene products of HIV

The *rev* gene of HIV codes for a small polypeptide of 116 amino acids which may act as a trans activating anti-repressor factor in viral replication Terwilliger *et al.*, 1986). Therefore drugs which inactivate and interfere with this protein may indirectly inhibit virus replication. It would also appear that the gene product of *tat* has an important control function, so making this gene produce a furthur important target for antiviral chemotherapy. Two further regulatory genes are *vif* and *nef* and again the protein products are, in theory, amenable to blockade by antiviral drugs. But a major problem is the absence of established methods for searching for drugs to inhibit these viral proteins. At present the most scientific method would appear to be the logical testing of overlapping short peptides, in a biological screen in cell culture, which might compete with important functional areas of the regulatory proteins. With X-ray crystallography of the respective proteins, which are all subjects of cloning experiments, it should be possible to design small molecules especially, as is most likely, an inhibitor is first found by chance. More specific in-vitro tests will need to be developed, perhaps to find compounds that inhibit direct binding of the regulatory proteins to proviral DNA.

But a particularly promising target for antiviral chemotherapy would appear to be the virus *pol* gene and its extremely important polypeptide gene products. The 5′ region of the retrovirus *pol* gene codes for a protease enzyme which cleaves *gag* and *gag-pol* polyproteins into functional proteins for incorporation into the mature infectious virion. An inhibitor of this protease enzyme would be expected to interfere with virus maturation (Pearl & Taylor, 1987). Certainly the HIV coded protease can be inhibited *in vitro* by pepstatin A, an aspartyl proteinase specific inhibitor (Katch *et al.*, 1987). The HIV coded protease is currently a favourite target because in-vitro tests of molecules able to inhibit specific proteolysis are relatively easy to design. As an alternative approach it may be possible to inhibit synthesis of the protease by suppression of the *gag* termination signal using specific oligonucleotides (see above).

A particularly important product of the virus is the endonuclease or integrase enzyme which must cut open the circularized HIV DNA prior to the integration step into human host cell chromosomal DNA. As noted above with the HIV protease enzyme, screening of overlapping short peptides of the correct endonuclease sequence is a possible way of finding inhibitors. In the absence of a precise biochemical screening test, it should be possible to design a biological screen searching for inhibitors of the *pol* polypeptides labelled intracellularly with S35 methionine and immunoprecipitated from lysates of virus infected cells.

Examination of the amino acid sequence of the *pol* gene of HIV and other retroviruses has identified a so-called zinc finger (Johnson *et al.*, 1986). Berg (1986) identified the separation of pairs of *his* and *cys* amino acids by 18 or so other amino acids as a zinc-binding motif. Such a configuration would chelate zinc, often found in zinc metalloenzymes via terdendate bonding with the *his* and *cys* amino acids. We have previously used chelation chemistry to devise and synthesize against other purported zinc metalloenzymes of influenza RNA replicase (Oxford & Perrin, 1974, 1977). Molecules such as methyl-isatin-thiosemicarbazones (Haase & Levinson, 1973) and acetyl pyridine thiosemicarbazone appear to inhibit influenza virus enzyme function by binding to the zinc in the metalloenzyme, thus forming a zinc-enzyme-inhibitor complex (Oxford & Perrin, 1974, 1977). The chelating agent D-penicillamine has been shown to have some HIV inhibitory effects, and could act in the same way. Most recently the chelating agent, imuthiol, has been shown to have clinical activity against HIV (Lang *et al.*, 1988).

Table IV. Sequence of amino acids of endonuclease of lentiviruses

HIV-2	RQVLFLEKIEPAQEE(H)EK (H)SNVKELSHKFGI PNLVARQIVNS(C)AQ(C)QQKGEAIHGQVNAELGTW
HIV-1	RKVLFLDGIDKAQDE(H)EK (H)SNWRAMASDFNL PPVVAKEIVAS(C)DK(C)QLKGEAMHGQLDCSPGIW
VISNA	TGMTWIENIPLAEEE(H)NKW(H)QDAVSLHLEFGI PRTAAEDIVQQ(C)DV(C)QENKMPST RGSNKRGIDHW

The so called 'zinc finger' is identified by the pairs of H and C amino acids separated by stretches of 23 or so amino acids. Zinc metalloenzyme function can be inhibited by chelation chemotherapy (Oxford & Perrin, 1977; Stradling *et al.*, 1986).

Inhibitors of intracellular processing of HIV proteins

Castanospermine is a plant alkaloid isolated from the seeds of the Australian chestnut tree *Castanospermium australe*. Like most anti-HIV inhibitors the discovery of the compound predates the time of isolation of HIV-1 (reviewed by Datema, Olofsson & Romero, 1987). The compound inhibits α-glucosidase I and therefore normal processing of the glycoprotein is disturbed and glucose residues are not removed. It is known that altered glycosylation can have profound effects on the functions of the protein and in the case of HIV-1 the properties of major glycoprotein gp120 are affected (Gruters *et al.*, 1987; Walker *et al.*, 1987). Since gp120 is known to have important catalytic functions in virus-host cell membrane fusion subsequent to attachment to the cellular CD4 cell receptor it is perhaps not surprising that virus induced syncytium formation is inhibited. There is evidence that sugar molecules cover exceptionally large areas of the HIV glycoprotein and hence changes could affect gp120 functions profoundly and to a greater degree than some normal cellular glycoproteins whose glycosylation patterns may be changed to a lesser extent. An additional observation to emerge from this study, relevant to methods of screening and searching for new antivirals, was that castanospermine had no effect on synthesis of HIV proteins in chronically infected cells, but nevertheless the released virus had a lower infectivity for fresh cultures of cells. Therefore the anti HIV activity of the compound could easily have been missed in the first in-vitro studies.

Inhibition of virus budding and changes in post budding morphology

The precise details of the birth or exit of new particles of HIV are not known. It is conceivable though that inhibitors such as amantadine or interferon could act at this stage (McClure, Marsh & Weiss, 1988). Moreover an interesting possibility for a new approach to antiviral chemotherapy of HIV is the post budding change in virus morphology that is triggered by unknown factors, both with retroviruses in general and the lentivirus HIV (Figure 2). At the present time a resort to random screening will be necessary to identify any molecule capable of preventing this morphological trigger, which presumably is necessary for the full infectivity of the virus to be attained.

Biological features of HIV which may be important in antiviral screening

Experience with other viruses, and with influenza in particular, has shown that the laboratory methodology is of vital importance in assessing the precise degree of antiviral activity of a potential inhibitor. Thus amantadine, a clinically effective inhibitor of influenza in epidemics, may show either marked or poor in-vitro inhibitory effects depending on the virus and cell system used in the laboratory test procedure (reviewed by Oxford & Galbraith, 1984). In particular, much-passaged or laboratory adapted viruses are poorly inhibited *in vitro* (Oxford & Galbraith, 1984). Also, differences in the degree of virus inhibition are noted with different antigenic subtypes of influenza. Analysis of in-vitro drug sensitivity of a number of field isolates of herpes simplex virus also uncovered a wide range of sensitivities to acyclovir (reviewed by Field, 1983).

Since sequence homology between some strains of HIV-1 virus is even less than between subtypes of influenza A, it is quite conceivable that a wide range of therapeutic indices may exist for any HIV inhibitor. Even more important is the distinct possibility that lead compounds might be missed if the biological screen uses

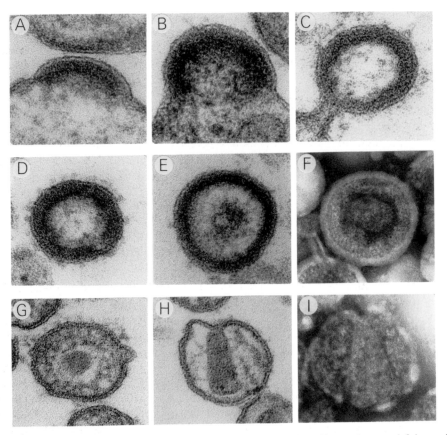

Figure 2. Electron micrographs illustrating development and maturation of human immunodeficiency virus. All micrographs are sectioned specimens except F and I which are negative staining specimens; all × 200,000. (Courtesy of Dr D. Hockley NIBSC, South Mimms, Potters Bar). A, B & C, Stages in budding of virus particles from the membrane of an infected cell. D, Newly-released, 'ring-like' immature virus particle. E, Central dense structure in immature particle. F, Negative staining showing immature virus particle. G, Further development of central dense nucleoid and loss of ring-like structure. H, Typical mature virus particle with elongated and tapering nucleoid. I, Negative staining of mature virus. The genetic control of the post-release change in morphology is not understood. The morphological switch does provide a unique opportunity for antiviral intervention.

unsuitable HIV isolates, perhaps with genetic and biological properties markedly different from the natural epidemic virus. In a final example of comparative virology, it has been shown that even single amino acid substitutions (Robertson *et al.*, 1987) in HA protein of epidemic influenza virus can influence the virulence (Oxford *et al.*, 1987) and antigenic structure (Oxford *et al.*, 1987) of the virus. Already some laboratory investigations have shown the varying biological properties of isolates of HIV-1 (Dahl, Martin & Miller, 1987). Therefore a range of susceptible cells including peripheral blood lymphocytes as well as 'transformed' cells such as CEM would be a minimum requirement in a biological screen for new antivirals together with two or three viruses of varying in-vitro biological characteristics.

Target groups for antiviral chemotherapy and conclusions

To our minds a most intriguing question is whether new anti-HIV compounds will emerge from random screening, as in the past, or whether the more logical and seemingly scientific method of custom synthesis will provide a major breakthrough. In either case an urgent requirement is the development of biochemical screening procedures, in addition to biological methods of viral cultivation, to aid in the search for inhibitors of regulatory gene function. Will drug resistance become a problem of some significance or, as in the case of influenza and herpes, will drug resistant variants be detectable but have little clinical significance? Already some studies have anticipated the potential problem of resistance and at the same time the relative toxicity of the nucleoside analogues by developing and comparing pairs of inhibitors with different functional abilities, and which may show synergistic activity (Hartshorn et al., 1987) and also, as with other microbial diseases, reduce the opportunity for drug resistant mutants to emerge. Even this approach must proceed with caution because of the first report of antagonism between two antivirals, ribavirin and zidovudine (Vogt et al., 1987). A particularly sensible combination of antivirals is zidovudine and immune stimulators such as interferon and several clinical studies of such combined therapy are in progress.

With the AIDS epidemic now spreading from the homosexual population into the wider community and infecting such diverse groups as haemophiliacs, pregnant or nursing mothers and children it is unlikely that a single antiviral compound will be equally useful in all groups. To give an example, in homosexuals often infected with a variety of other viruses, stimulation of HIV latency may be enhanced and the most effective antiviral might be the compound with a broad spectrum of antiviral activity to include HIV and herpes viruses. The latter is most important as there is persuasive evidence that herpes gene products can cause activation of the HIV provirus DNA.

Our own interest is the search for, and clinical testing of, virus inhibitory molecules with very low or absent side effects which can be used in asymptomatic persons rather than in AIDS patients per se. Of course, there is some evidence that low dose zidovudine may have beneficial effects during this asymptomatic period (de Wolf et al., 1988). But we are investigating the potential clinical, immunological and antiviral effects of other compounds such as rifabutin, an inhibitor of viral RT, as a possible new member of a generation of specific but less toxic anti-HIV inhibitors (Anand et al., 1986).

Undoubtedly the task of finding a relatively non toxic inhibitor of such a diverse group of viruses as the human lentiviruses (including HIV-2, and HTLV-I and II) is a formidable one. It is still possible that this search for a specific inhibitor will fail, or at least fall very short of our expectations, but it will be an exciting and challenging period for antiviral chemotherapists who will occupy a pivotal role in attempts to control the AIDS epidemic.

Acknowledgements

We would like to thank Dr D. Hockley for his electron micrographs of budding of HIV and Maureen Measure for typing the manuscript.

References

Anand, R., Moore, J., Fedrino, P., Curran, J. & Srinavasan, A. (1986). Rifabutin inhibits HTLV-III. *Lancet* i, 97–8.

Balzarini, J., Kang, G.-J., Dalal, M., Herdewijn, P., de Clercq, E., Broder, S. et al. (1987). The anti-HTLV-III (Anti-HIV) and cytoxic activity of 2′,3′-didehydro-2′,3′-dideoxyribonucleosides: A comparison with their parental 2′,3′-dideoxyribonucleosides. *Molecular Pharmacology* **32**, 162–7.

Barré-Sinoussi, F., Chermann, J. C., Rey, F., Nugeyre, M. J., Chamaret, S., Gruest, J. *et al.* (1983). Isolation of T lymphotropic retrovirus from a patient at risk for acquired immune deficiency syndrome (AIDS). *Science* **220**, 868–70.

Bauer, D. J. (1985). A history of the discovery and clinical application of antiviral drugs. *British Medical Bulletin* **41**, 309–14.

Berg, J. M. (1986). Potential metal-binding domains in nucleic acid binding proteins. *Science* **232**, 485–7.

Choppin, P. W., Richardson, C. D. & Scheid, A. (1983). Analogues of viral polypeptides which specifically inhibit viral replication. In *Problems of Antiviral Therapy* (Stuart-Harris, C. H. & Oxford, J. S., Eds), Academic Press, London.

Coen, D. M., Chiou, H. C. & Gibbs, J. S. (1986). Molecular genetics of antiviral chemotherapy of herpes viruses. In *Human Herpesvirus Infections* (Lopez, C. & Roizman, B. Eds), pp. 117–8. Raven Press, New York.

Colman, P. M., Laver, W. G., Varghese, J. N., Baker, A. T., Tulloch, P. A., Air, G. M. *et al.* (1987). Three dimensional structure of a complex of antibody with influenza neuraminidase. *Nature* **326**, 358–63.

Dahl, K., Martin, K. & Miller, G. (1987). Differences among human immunodeficiency virus strains in their capacities to induce cytolysis or persistent infection of a lymphoblastoid cell line immortalized by Epstein-Barr virus. *Journal of Virology* **61**, 1602–8.

Datema, R., Olofsson, S. & Romero, P. A. (1987). Inhibition of protein glycosylation and glycoprotein processing in viral systems. *Pharmacology and Therapeutics* **33**, 221–86.

De Clercq E. (1988). Targets and potential drugs for the treatment of AIDS. *Journal of Antimicrobial Chemotherapy* **23**, *Suppl. A,* 35–46.

De Clercq, E., Holy, A., Rosenberg, I., Sakuma, T., Balzarini, J. & Maudgal, P. C. (1986). A novel selective broad spectrum anti-DNA virus agent. *Nature* **323**, 464–7.

De Wolf, F., Goudsmit, J., De Gans, J., Coutinho, R. A., Lange, J. M. A., Cload, P. *et al.* (1988). Effect of Zidovudine on serum human immunodeficiency virus antigen levels in symptom free subjects. *Lancet i,* 373–8.

Dormont, D. *et al.* (1985). Inhibition of RNA dependent DNA polymerase of AIDS and AIDS retroviruses by NPA–23. *Annals Institut Pasteur* **136**, 75–83.

Dutia, B. N., Frame, M. C., Subak-Sharpe, J. M., Clark, W. N. & Marsden, M. S. (1986). Specific inhibition of herpes virus ribonucleotide reductase by synthetic peptides. *Nature* **321**, 439–41.

Eiklid, K., Olsnes, S. & Pihl, A. (1980). Entry of lethal doses of abrin, ricin and modeccin into the cytosol of HeLa Cells. *Experimental Cell Research* **126**, 321–6.

Field, H. J. (1983). The problem of drug induced resistance in viruses. In *Problems of Antiviral Therapy,* (Stuart-Harris, C. H. & Oxford, J. S., Eds), pp. 71–101. Academic Press, London.

Fisch, M. A., Richman, D. D., Grieco, M. H., Gottliels, M. S., Volberding, P. A., Laskin, O. L. *et al.,* (1987). The efficacy of azidothymidine (AZT) in the treatment of patients with AIDS or AIDS related complex—a double blind placebo controlled trial. *New England Journal of Medicine* **317**, 185–91.

Geyson, H. M., Rodda, S. J., Mason, T. J., Tribbick, G. & Schoofs, P. G. (1987). Strategies for epitope analysis using peptide synthesis. *Journal of Immunological Methods* **102**, 259.

Gruters, R. A., Neefjes, J. J., Tersmette, M., de Goede, R. E. Y., Tulp, A., Huisman, M. G. *et al.* (1987). Interference with HIV-induced syncytium formation and viral infectivity by inhibitors of trimming glucosidase. *Nature* **330**, 74–7.

Hartshorn, K. L., Vogt, M. W., Chou, T.-C., Blumberg, R. S., Byington, R., Schooley, R. T. *et al.* (1987). Synergistic inhibition of human immunodeficiency virus *in vitro* by azidothymidine and recombinant alpha A interferon. *Antimicrobial Agents and Chemotherapy* **31**, 168–72.

Haase, A. T. & Levinson, W. (1973). Inhibition of RNA slow viruses by thiosemicarbazones. *Biochemical and Biophysical Research Communications* **51**, 875–80.

Hirsch, M. S. (1988). Azidothymidine. *Journal of Infectious Diseases* **157**, 427–31.

Ho, D. D., Hartshorn, K. L., Rota, T. R., Andrews, C. A., Schooley, R. T. & Hirsch, M. S. (1985). Recombinant human interferon alfa-A suppresses HTLV-III replication *in vitro*. *Lancet i,* 602–4.

Hussey, R. E., Richardson, N. E., Kowalski, M., Brown, N. R., Chang, M.-C., Siliciano, R. F.

et al. (1988). A soluble CD4 protein selectively inhibits HIV replication and syncytium formation. *Nature* **331**, 78–84.

Jasmin, C. *et al.* (1973). In vitro effects of silicotungstate on some RNA viruses. *Biomedicine* **18**, 319–27.

Johnson, M. S., McClure, M. A., Feng, D.-F. & Doolittle, R. F. (1986). Computer analysis of retroviral pol genes: Assignment of enzymatic functions to specific sequences and homologies with nonviral enzymes. *Proceedings of the National Academy of Science, USA* **83**, 7648–52.

Katch, I., Yasunaga, T., Ikawa, Y. & Yoshinaka, Y. (1987). Inhibition of retroviral protease activity by an aspartyl proteinase inhibitor. *Nature* **329**, 654–6.

Larder, B., Purifoy, D., Powell, K. & Darby, G. (1987). AIDS virus reverse transcriptase defined by high level expression in *Escherichia coli*. *EMBO Journal* **6**, 3133–7.

Lin, T.-S., Schinazi, R. F. & Prusoff, W. H. (1987). Potent and selective *in vitro* activity of 3'-deoxythymidin-2'-ene (3'-deoxy-2',3'didehydrothymidine) against human immunodeficiency virus). *Biochemical Pharmacology* **36**, 2713–8.

Minor, P. D. (1988). Strategies for the development of vaccines against HIV. *Journal of Antimicrobial Chemotherapy* **23**, Suppl. A, 55–62.

Maddon, P. J., Dalgleish, A. G., McDougal, J. S., Clapham, P. R., Weiss, R. A. & Axel, R. (1986). The T4 gene encodes the AIDS virus receptor and is expressed in the immune system and the brain. *Cell* **47**, 333–48.

Matsukura, M., Shinozuka, K., Zon, G., Mitsuya, H., Reitz, M., Cohen, J. S. *et al.* (1987). Phosphorothioate analogs of oligodeoxynucleotides: inhibitors of replication and cytopathic effects of human immunodeficiency virus. *Proceedings of the National Academy of Science, USA* **84**, 7706–10.

McClure, M. O., Marsh, M. & Weiss, R. A. (1988). Human immunodeficiency virus infection of CD4-bearing cells occurs by a pH-independent mechanism. *EMBO Journal* **7**, 513–8.

McCormick, J. B., Mitchell, S. W., Getchell, J. P. & Hicks, D. R. (1984). Ribavirin suppresses replication of lymphadenopathy associated virus in cultures of human adult lymphocytes. *Lancet ii*, 1367–9.

McDaniel, H. R. & McAnalley, B. H. (1987). Evaluation of polymannoacetate in the treatment of AIDS. *Clinical Research* **35**, 483.

Melton, D. A. (1985). Injected anti-sense RNAs specifically block messenger RNA translation *in vivo*. *Proceedings of the National Academy of Science, USA* **82**, 144–8.

Mitsuya, H., Popovic M., Tarchoan, R., Matsushita, S., Gallo, R. C. & Broder, S. (1984). Suramin protection of T cells *in vitro* against infecting and cytopathic effect of HTLV-III. *Science* **226**, 172–4.

Mitsuya, H. & Broder, S. (1986). Inhibition of the *in vitro* infectivity and cytopathic effect of human T-lymphotrophic virus type III/lymphadenopathy-associated virus (HTLV-III/LAV) by 2',3'-dideoxynucleosides. *Proceedings of the National Academy of Sciences, USA* **83**, 1911–5.

Mitsuya, H. & Broder, S. (1987). Strategies for antiviral therapy in AIDS. *Nature* **325**, 773–8.

Mitsuya, H., Jarrett, R. F., Matsukura, M., Veronese, F. D. M., Sarngadharan, M. G., Johns, D. G. *et al.* (1987). Long-term inhibition of human T-lymphotropic virus type III/lymphadenopathy-associated virus (human immunodeficiency virus) DNA synthesis and RNA expression in T-cells protected by 2',3'-dideoxynucleosides *in vitro*. *Proceedings of the National Academy of Science, USA* **84**, 2033–7.

Nabel, G. J., Rice, S. A. Knipe, D. M. & Baltimore, D. (1988). Alternative mechanisms for activation of human immunodeficiency virus enhancer in T-cells. *Science* **239**, 1299–301.

Oberg, B. (1986). Antiviral chemotherapy against HTLV-III/LAV infections. *Journal of Antimicrobial Chemotherapy* **17**, 549–52.

Oxford, J. S. & Perrin, D. D. (1974). Inhibition of the particle associated RNA dependent RNA polymerase activity of influenza virus by chelating agents. *Journal of General Virology* **23**, 59–71.

Oxford, J. S. & Perrin, D. D. (1977). Influenza RNA transcriptase inhibitors. Studies *in vitro* and *in vivo*. *Annals of the New York Academy of Sciences* **284**, 613–23.

Oxford, J. S. & Galbraith, A. (1984). Anti influenza virus activity of amantadine. (Shugar, D., Ed.), pp. 160–224. In *Viral Chemotherapy*, Vol. 1, Pergamon Press, Oxford.

Oxford, J. S. & Oberg, B. (1985). *Conquest of Viral Disease: a Topical Review of Antivirals and Vaccines*, p. 715. Elsevier Biomedical Press, Amsterdam.

Oxford, J. S., Corcoran, T., Knott, R., Bates, J., Bartholomei, O. & Major, D. (1987). Serological studies of influenza A (HINI) viruses cultivated in eggs or in a canine kidney cell line (MDCK). *Bulletin WHO* **65**, 181–7.

Pearl, L. H. & Taylor, W. R. (1987). A structural model for the retroviral proteases. *Nature* **329**, 351–4.

Pert, C. O., Hill, J. M., Ruff, M. R., Berman, R. M., Robey, W. G., Arthur, L. O. *et al.* (1986). Octapeptides deduced from the neuropeptide receptor-like pattern of antigen CD4+ in brain potently inhibit human immunodeficiency virus receptor binding and T cell infectivity. *Proceedings of National Academy of Sciences, USA* **83**, 8254–6.

Richman, D. D. Fischl, M. A., Grieco, M. H., Gottliels, M. S., Volberding, P. A., Laskin. O. L. *et al.* (1987) The toxicity of azidothymidine (AZT) in the treatment of patients with AIDS and AIDS related complex—a double blind placebo controlled trial. *New England Journal of Medicine* **317**, 192–7.

Robertson, J. S., Bootman, J. S., Newman, R., Oxford, J. S., Daniels, R. S., Webster, R. G. *et al.* (1987). Structure changes in the haemoglutin in which accompany egg adaptation of an influenza A (HINI) virus. *Virology* **160**, 31–7.

Rozenbaum, W., Dormont, D., Spire, B., Vilmer, E., Gentilini, M., Griscelli, C. *et al.* (1985). Autimoniotungistenate (MPA23) treatment of three patients with AIDS and one with prodrome *Lancet i*, 450–1.

Sarin, P. S., Gallo, R. C., Scheer, D. I., Crews, F. & Lippa, A. S. (1985). Effects of AL-721 on HTLV-III infectivity *in vitro*. *New England Journal of Medicine* **313**, 1289–90.

Sarin, P. (1987). Suppression of AIDS virus replication *in vivo* by D penicillamine. *International Conference on AIDS, Washington, (Abstract)*, p. 24.

Schuster, M., Cohn, J. & McMeeking, A. (1986). Disinfection for HTLV-III halogenated soaps. *Journal of the American Medical Association* **255**, 2290–1.

Smith, T. J., Kremer, M. J., Luo, M., Vriend, G., Arnold, E., Kamer, G. *et al.* (1986). The site of attachment of human rhinovirus 14 for antiviral agents that inhibit uncoating. *Science* **233**, 1286–93.

Spire, B., Barré-Sinoussi, F., Montognier, L. & Chermann, J. C. (1984). Inactivation of lymphadenopathy associated virus by chemical disinfectants. *Lancet ii*, 899–901.

Stein, B. S., Gowda, S. D., Lifson, J. D., Penhallow, R. C., Bensch, K. G. & Englemon, E. G. (1987). pH independent HIV entry into CD4-positive T cells via virus envelope fusion to the plasma membrane. *Cell* **49**, 659–68.

Stradling, G. N., Stather, J. W., Gray, S. A., Moody, J. C., Ellender, M. & Hodgson, A. (1986). Efficacies of LICAM(C) and DTPA for the decorporation of inhaled transportable forms of plutonium and americium from the rat. *Human Toxicology* **5**, 77–84.

Stuart-Harris, C. H., Schild, G. C. & Oxford, J. S. (1985). *Influenza, the Virus and the Disease*. Edward Arnold, London.

Terwilliger, E., Sodroski, J. G., Rosen, C. A. & Haseltine, W. A. (1986). Effects of mutations within the 3' orf open reading frame region of human T-cell lymphotropic virus type III (HTLV-III/LAV) on replication and cytopathogenicity. *Journal of Virology* **60**, 754–60.

Thuong, N. T., Asseline, U., Roig, V., Takasugi, M. & Helene, C. (1987). Oligo (-deoxy-nucleotide)s covalently linked to intercalating agents; Differential binding to ribo- and deoxy-ribopolynucleotides and stability towards nuclease digestion. *Proceedings of the National Academy of Sciences, USA* **84**, 5129–33.

Toulmé, J. J., Krisch, H. M., Loreau, N., Thuong, N. T. & Hélène, C. (1986). Specific inhibition of mRNA translation by complementary oligonucleotides covalently linked to intercalating agents. *Proceedings of the National Academy of Science, USA* **83**, 1227–31.

Uhlenbeck, O. C. (1987). A small catalytic oligoribonucleotide. *Nature* **328**, 596–600.

Uhr, J. W. (1984). American Association of Immunologists-Presidential address—Immunotoxins: harnessing nature's poisons. *Journal of Immunology* **133**, ii–ix.

Vogt, M. W., Hartshorn, K. L., Furman, P. A. Chou, T.-C., Fyfe, J. A. Coleman, L. A. *et al.* (1987). Ribavirin antagonizes the effect of azidothymidine on HIV replication. *Science* **235**, 1376–9.

Walker, B. D., Kowalski, M., Goh, W. C., Kozarsky, K., Krieger, M., Rosen, C. *et al.* (1987).

Inhibition of human immunodeficiency virus syncytium formation and virus relication by castanospermine. *Proceedings of the National Academy of Sciences, USA* **84,** 8120–4.

Weber, J. (1988). The biology and epidemiology of HIV infections. *Journal of Antimicrobial Chemotherapy* **23,** Suppl. A, 1–7.

Wilson, I. A., Skehel, J. J. & Wiley, D. C. (1981). The structure of the haemagglutinin membrane glycoprotein of influenza virus at 3 Å resolution. *Nature* **298,** 366–73.

Yarchoan, R. & Broder, S. (1987). Development of antiretroviral therapy for the acquired immunodeficiency syndrome and related disorders: A progress report. *New England Journal of Medicine* **316,** 557–64.

Yarchoan, R., Klecher, R. W., Weinhold, K. J., Markham, P. D., Lyerly, H. J., Durack, D. T. *et al.* (1986). Administration of 3′-azido-3′-deoxythymidine, an inhibitor of HTLV-III/LAV replication, to patients with AIDS or AIDS-related complex. *Lancet i,* 575–80.

Yarchoan, R., Thomas, R. V., Allain, J.-P., McAtee, N., Dubinsky, R. Mitsuya, H. *et al.* (1988). Phase 1 studies of 2′,3′dideoxycytidine in severe human immunodeficiency virus infection as a single agent and alternating with zidovudine (AZT). *Lancet i,* 76–81.

Zamecnik, P. C. & Stephenson, M. L. (1977). Inhibition of Rous sarcoma virus replication and cell transformation by a specific oligodeoxynucleotide. *Proceedings of the National Academy of Science, USA* **65,** 280–4.

Zamecnik, P. C., Goodchild, J., Taguchi, Y. & Sarin, P. S. (1986). Inhibition of replication and expression of human T cell lymphotropic virus type III in cultured cells by exogenous synthetic oligonucleotides complementary to viral RNA. *Proceedings of the National Academy of Science, USA* **83,** 4143–6.

Journal of Antimicrobial Chemotherapy (1989) **23**, Suppl. A, 29–34

The antiviral activity of dideoxycytidine

D. J. Jeffries

Division of Virology, St. Mary's Hospital Medical School, Paddington, London W2 1PG, UK

2′,3′-Dideoxycytidine (ddc) is a 2′,3′-dideoxypyrimidine nucleotide which has been shown to be active against human immunodeficiency virus type 1 (HIV-1) in cell cultures. This article reviews some of the laboratory studies with this antiviral compound, and available pharmacokinetic and toxicity data from phase 1 studies of ddc alone and in alternation with zidovudine in patients with AIDS and ARC. Though ddc has potent activity against HIV-1 *in vitro*, serious toxic effects seen in phase 1 studies warrant continuation of trials to explore lower dosage regimens, alternation with zidovudine and intermittent therapy.

Preclinical studies of dideoxycytidine

Mitsuya & Broder (1986) demonstrated that, with the ribose moiety of the molecule in a 2′,3′-dideoxy configuration, every purine (adenosine, guanosine and inosine) and pyrimidine (cytidine and thymidine) nucleoside tested suppressed HIV-1 replication. In comparative studies 2′,3′-dideoxycytidine (ddc) (Figure 1) was the most active, on a molar basis, of the analogues tested. The present review will consider some of the laboratory and clinical effects of this antiviral compound. Initial laboratory studies of ddc were performed in ATH8 cells, an OKT4+(CD4+) T cell clone immortalized by infection with human T lymphotropic virus type 1 (HTLV-1). These cells do not produce HTLV-1 and they are permissive for HIV-1 infection with marked sensitivity to the cytopathic effect of the virus (cell death). Uninfected ATH8 cells increased approximately three-fold in number after five days in culture while, in contrast, more than 98% of cells were killed following infection with HIV-1 (HTLV-3B strain-2000

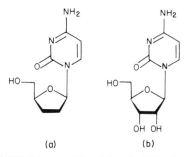

(a) (b)

Figure 1. Chemical structure of 2′,3′-dideoxycytidine (a) and relationship to cytidine (b).

0305–7453/89/23A029 + 06 \$02.00/0

virus particles per cell). Infected cells were fully protected from the cytopathic effect of the virus at concentrations of 0·5 µmol or more, with partial protection at 0·05 and 0·1 µmol. Inhibition of replication of uninfected ATH8 cells by ddc was observed at concentrations greater than 10 µmol. Similar results were obtained when ATH8 cells were infected with HIV-1 and treated with ddc for seven and ten days.

The protective effect of ddc was confirmed in TM3 cells, a clone of normal helper/inducer T cells, that were co-cultured with irradiated H9/HTLV-3B infected cells. Infected cultures showed no cytopathic effect after 14 days in the presence of a single concentration (5 µmol) of ddc that did not inhibit the replication of uninfected cells (Mitsuya & Broder, 1986). Inhibition of viral p24 antigen production was demonstrated in H9 cells, a clone of CD4+ T lymphoblastoid cells which is permissive for HIV-1 replication but is partly resistant to its cytopathic effects (Popovic et al., 1984). Production of p24 antigen was completely suppressed over the experimental period (8–10 days) by ddc concentrations of 1·0 µmol or greater and partially suppressed by 0·1 µmol.

Previous studies of the effect of nucleoside analogues on other viruses have shown variations in sensitivity in different cell types. This has been correlated with the availability of phosphorylating enzymes. Thus, Richman et al. (1987a) reported that dideoxynucleotides, including ddc, were ineffective in inhibiting HIV-1 replication in monocyte-derived macrophages. This lack of activity was associated with reduced nucleoside kinase activity in cultured macrophages when compared to lymphocytes. It remains to be seen, however, whether these cells are representative of macrophages present in vivo. Human macrophages have been reported to lack thymidine kinase activity and to release deoxypyrimidines extracellularly (Vercammen-Grandjean et al., 1981) and Cooney et al. (1986), in a study of various cell types, found lack of phosphorylation of ddc in a macrophage-derived cell line (p388/AAC). These findings may be of importance in assessing the likely effect of ddc and other nucleotide analogues in controlling HIV-1 infection in vivo.

Mechanism of antiviral action of ddc

The exact mechanism of action of ddc remains unknown but it is believed to remain inactive until it is metabolized to the 5′-triphosphate by host cell enzymes. Phosphorylation to the mono-, di, and tri-phosphates occurs in infected and uninfected cells and the nucleoside 5′-triphosphate is thought to act as a substrate for HIV-1 reverse transcriptase with subsequent inhibition of formation of proviral DNA. Phosphorylation of ddc, and its antiviral activity in vitro, are inhibited by the presence of a five molar excess of 2′-deoxycytidine, indicating competitive inhibition as substrates for the reverse transcriptase. Analysis of the phosphorylated derivatives of ddc, in infected and uninfected cells, has revealed the formation of an additional metabolite which has been identified tentatively as a dideoxycytidine diphosphate-choline adduct (Cooney et al., 1986); the significance of this finding awaits clarification. Starnes & Cheng (1987) examined the phosphorylation of ddc in uninfected cells of human origin (Molt 4) and found that the extent of intracellular accumulation of the compound was dependent on the concentration in the extracellular medium. The phosphorylated metabolites were present in constant proportions and declined when ddc was removed from the medium.

Three DNA polymerases are involved in normal cell growth. DNA polymerase alpha is the principal enzyme responsible for nuclear DNA replication, beta is thought to be involved in nuclear DNA repair processes, and gamma generates mitochondrial DNA. These enzymes show different degrees of sensitivity to the action of ddc; the alpha DNA polymerase (inhibition constant K_i, 110 μmol) is considerably less sensitive than the beta and gamma polymerases (K_i, 2·6 and 0·016 respectively) (Starnes & Cheng, 1987).

Studies of ddc in HIV-1 infected ATH8 cells *in vitro* have revealed inhibition of viral DNA synthesis resulting from DNA chain termination (Mitsuya *et al.*, 1987). The 5′-triphosphate of ddc acted as a substrate for HIV-1 reverse transcriptase with elongation of the DNA chain by one residue followed by failure to form further 5′3′-phospho-diester linkages.

Clinical studies with ddc

Preliminary pharmacokinetic and toxicity data have been obtained from a phase 1 study of ddc in patients with AIDS and ARC. The results of this study involving different dosage regimens of ddc alone, and limited data of its use in a weekly alternating schedule with zidovudine have been reported by Yarchoan *et al.* (1988).

Pharmacokinetics

The oral bio-availability of ddc appears to be good with 70–80% of the administered dose appearing in the circulation. Animal studies have suggested, however, that absorption may be affected by food (Kelley *et al.*, 1987). The average elimination half-life in humans is 1·2 h and, in animal experiments, more than 90% of the drug has been recovered unchanged in the urine with some conversion (in monkeys) to dideoxyuridine. In the phase 1 studies, analysis of cerebrospinal fluid was performed on five patients and measurable amounts of ddc were detected 2–3·5 h after intravenous infusion. These single time point studies cannot be used to assess the extent of penetration of the blood-brain barrier but cerebrospinal fluid : plasma ratios varied from 9–37%.

Safety/tolerance studies

Twenty patients with AIDS or ARC were enrolled in a study at the National Cancer Institute in the United States. Following a single intravenous dose of ddc, followed by a single oral dose, patients received two weeks of intravenous administration and then four weeks of oral treatment. Many of the patients continued on oral therapy after this regimen. The following dosage schedules were used: 0·03 mg/kg eight-hourly, 0·03 mg/kg four-hourly, 0·06 mg/kg four-hourly, 0·09 mg/kg four-hourly and 0·25 mg/kg eight-hourly.

Marked toxicity was seen from use of ddc in these patients of which the most important effects were painful peripheral neuropathy with a' glove-stocking distribution, neutropenia and thrombocytopenia. A transient complex of toxic side-effects was common during initial therapy and included skin rashes, malaise, fever, aphthous mouth ulceration and, to a lesser extent, arthralgia, ankle oedema, nail changes and diarrhoea. There was considerable variation in the severity and expression of this early toxicity and, in each of the seven cases in whom ddc therapy was continued despite these effects, the symptoms and signs subsided.

Painful peripheral neuropathy occurred after eight to twelve weeks in ten of the patients who continued on the drug after the initial six weeks of therapy and was prominent even in those receiving the lowest doses. It usually began with numbness, tingling and burning of the soles of the feet and worsened with continued therapy. Later, patients exhibited loss of light touch and temperature, vibratory and proprioceptive sensation and, in severe cases, numbness, weakness and absent ankle jerks developed. Electrophysiological studies were consistent with axonal degeneration and it has been noted that these neurological changes are similar to the peripheral neuropathy seen in severe AIDS. The neuropathy worsened for up to five weeks after cessation of treatment and then most patients showed gradual clinical and electromyographical improvement.

Some patients who received lower doses of the drug became mildly thrombocytopenic but this subsided despite continuation of therapy. In contrast, however, in three individuals on the highest doses thrombocytopenia and neutropenia were dose-limiting side effects. Marrow examination showed erythroblastic vacuolization in two of these patients although megaloblastic change was not prominent and they did not show the increases in red-cell mean corpuscular volume observed in patients receiving zidovudine.

Clinical, virological and immunological effects

No meaningful assessment of clinical efficacy can be obtained from these studies in view of the small numbers of patients, the short duration of treatment and the severe toxicity reactions. Yarchoan et al. (1988) have shown details of serum p24 antigen levels in patients receiving different dosage regimes of ddc but there is no clear indication of a virological effect. Claims of an early decline of p24 antigen are unconvincing in the absence of adequate baseline or control values. Similarly, there was no observed benefit on the levels of circulating CD4 + lymphocytes within the six week assessment period.

Alternating ddc and zidovudine therapy

On the basis of an assessment that ddc had some activity in vivo against HIV-1, and also as it showed a different toxicity profile to zidovudine, six patients were entered into a study of alternating therapy. Zidovudine (200 mg every 4 h for seven days) was alternated with ddc (0·03 mg/kg every 4 h for seven days). One patient was withdrawn after two weeks as he developed neutropenia and a sepsis-like picture, and Mycobacterium avium was isolated from numerous blood cultures. The other five patients had negligible or transient drug-related symptoms during the nine week follow-up period and four elected to continue on the regimen. The fifth had ddc-associated arthralgia during weeks six to eight and decided to stop. One patient, who had been on the earlier ddc study developed burning of the feet during his first week on zidovudine. This was considered to be a late effect of ddc and it subsided as he continued on the alternating regimen (it recurred again in mild form at 12 weeks). The remaining three patients completed 28 weeks of therapy without neuropathic symptoms and an overall mean increase of 5·4 fl in their red-cell mean corpuscular volume during the first nine weeks was less than might have been expected with zidovudine given as a single agent (Richman *et al.*, 1987*b*; Yarchoan & Broder, 1987).

Conclusions

Laboratory studies showed that ddc has potent activity against HIV-1. The chemotherapeutic index is, however, less than that of zidovudine and this is reflected in the serious toxic effects seen in the phase 1 studies. Further clinical trials are in progress including the continuation of treatment in alternation with zidovudine, exploration of lower dosage schedules, and intermittent therapy. It may be important to note that ddc acts via a different phosphokinase system to zidovudine and this could be a significant determinant in selecting drug combinations or alternating therapies in the future, particularly if mutant viruses, resistant to zidovudine, start to emerge. It remains to be seen whether, by careful selection of dosage regimens, the powerful anti-retroviral effect of ddc can be harnessed to allow the long-term therapy of HIV-1 infected individuals with this drug alone. It is also open to question whether the low oral doses of ddc which are likely to be necessary to avoid toxicity will be adequate to allow a therapeutic concentration to enter the central nervous system.

References

Cooney, D. A., Dalal, M., Mitsuya, H., McMahon, J. B., Nadkarni, M., Balzarni, J. *et al.* (1986). Initial studies on the cellular pharmacology of 2′,3′-dideoxycytidine, an inhibitor of HTLV-III infectivity. *Biochemical Pharmacology* **35**, 2065–68.

Kelley, J. A., Litterst, C. L., Roth, J. S., Vistica, D. T., Poplack, D. G., Cooney, D. A. *et al.* (1987). The disposition and metabolism of 2′,3′-dideoxycytidine, an in vitro inhibitor of HTLV-1 infectivity, in mice and monkeys. *Drug Metabolism and Disposition* **15**, 595–601.

Mitsuya, H. & Broder, S. (1986). Inhibition of the *in vitro* infectivity and cytopathic effect of human T-lymphotropic virus type III/lymphadenopathy-associated virus (HTLV-III/LAV) by 2′,3′-dideoxynucleotides. *Proceedings of the National Academy of Sciences USA* **83**, 1911–5.

Mitsuya, H., Jarrett, R. F., Matsukura, M., Di Marzo Veronese, F., De Vico, A. L., Sarngadharan, M. G. *et al.* (1987). Long-term inhibition of human T-lymphotropic virus type III/lymphadenopathy associated virus (human immunodeficiency virus) DNA synthesis and RNA expression in T cells protected by 2′,3′-dideoxynucleosides *in vitro*. *Proceedings of the National Academy of Sciences USA* **84**, 2033–7.

Popovic, M., Sarngadharan, S. Z., Read, E. & Gallo, R. C. (1984). Detection, isolation and continuous production of cytopathic retroviruses (HTLV-III) from patients with AIDS and pre-AIDS. *Science* **224**, 497–500.

Richman, D. D., Fischl, M. A., Grieco, M. H., Gottlieb, M. S., Volberding, P. A., Laskin, O. C. *et al.* (1987*a*). The toxicity of azidothymidine (AZT) in the treatment of patients with AIDS and AIDS-related complex. A double-blind placebo-controlled trial. *New England Journal of Medicine* **317**, 192–7.

Richman, D. D., Kornbluth, R. S. & Carson, D. A. (1987*b*). Failure of dideoxynucleosides to inhibit human immunodeficiency virus replication in cultured human macrophages. *Journal of Experimental Medicine* **166**, 1144–9.

Starnes, M. C. & Cheng, Y. (1987). Cellular metabolism of 2′,3′-dideoxycytidine, a compound active against human immunodeficiency virus *in vitro*. *Journal of Biological Chemistry* **262**, 988–91.

Vercammen-Grandjean, A. R., Arnould, A., Libert, P., Ewalenko, P. & Lejeune, F. (1981). Production of the effector molecule thymidine by human lung alveolar macrophages. *European Journal of Cancer and Oncology* **20**, 1543–6.

Yarchoan, R. & Broder, S. (1987). Development of antiretroviral therapy for the acquired immunodeficiency syndrome and related disorders. *New England Journal of Medicine* **316,** 557–64.

Yarchoan, R., Perno, C. F., Thomas, R. V., Klecker, R. W., Allain, J-P., Wills, R. J. *et al.* (1988). Phase 1 studies of 2′,3′-dideoxycytidine in severe human immunodeficiency virus infection as a single agent and alternating with zidovudine (AZT). *Lancet i,* 76–80.

Journal of Antimicrobial Chemotherapy (1989) **23**, *Suppl. A*, 35–46

Potential drugs for the treatment of AIDS

Erik De Clercq

*Rega Institute for Medical Research, Katholieke Universiteit Leuven,
Minderbroedersstraat 10, B-3000 Leuven, Belgium*

From our investigations the following compounds have emerged as particularly potent and selective inhibitors of HIV replication: sulphated polysaccharides (i.e. heparin, dextran sulphate, pentosan polysulphate), dideoxynucleoside analogues such as the 3'-azido- and 3'-fluoro-substituted 2',3'-dideoxyribosides of both purines (i.e. guanine, 2,6-diaminopurine) and pyrimidines (i.e. uracil, thymine), and the 9-(2-phosphonylmethoxyethyl) derivatives of adenine, 2-monoaminopurine and 2,6-diaminopurine. All these compounds yield great promise for the treatment of retrovirus infections in humans. Whereas the sulphated polysaccharides interfere with the virus adsorption process, the nucleoside analogues (following intracellular phosphorylation to their 5'-triphosphate) appear to be targeted at the reverse transcriptase.

Introduction

The replicative cycle of human immunodeficiency virus (HIV) encompasses a number of steps that could be considered as adequate targets for antiviral agents: virus adsorption and penetration, uncoating of the viral RNA genome, reverse transcription of the viral RNA to DNA, followed by duplication of the latter to double-stranded DNA, circularization and integration of the proviral DNA in the cellular genome, transcription of the proviral DNA to viral mRNA, translation of the latter to viral proteins, processing (proteolytic cleavage, glycosylation and myristylation) of the viral proteins, and, finally, assembly and release (budding) of the new virus particles.

The virus replication steps that have received most attention as targets for antiviral chemotherapy are: (i) virus adsorption to the cell membrane, which is based on an interaction of the viral envelope glycoprotein gp 120 with the cellular CD4 receptor; (ii) reverse transcription of the viral RNA to DNA, which requires the help of the virus-associated reverse transcriptase (RT); this enzyme transcribes the single-stranded viral RNA genome to an RNA-DNA hybrid, the RNA part of which is then degraded by RNase H; (iii) the transcription of proviral DNA to viral mRNA, which is activated by the *trans*-acting transcriptional (TAT) activator, itself a viral product that stimulates the transcription of the proviral DNA genome starting from the TAT recognition (TAR) site in the 5'-LTR (long terminal repeat) region; (iv) proteolytic cleavage of the viral GAG-POL (group-specific antigen/polymerase) polyprotein by the viral protease (PRO) into the separate GAG proteins (GAG 17, GAG 24, GAG 15) and POL proteins, PRO, RT and END (endonuclease, integrase), the latter being required for integration of proviral DNA into cellular DNA; and, finally; (v) the glycosylation process of the viral glycoproteins which starts with the initial core

0305–7453/89/23A035 + 12 $02.00/0

glycosylation, then requires trimming by glucosidases and mannosidases before proceeding on to terminal glycosylation.

Among the most potent and selective inhibitors of HIV replication described to date are the sulphated polysaccharides which are apparently targeted at the virus adsorption process, and the dideoxynucleoside analogues which are targeted at the reverse transcription step (after their conversion to the 5′-triphosphate derivatives). Akin to the dideoxynucleoside analogues, the phosphonylmethoxyethyl purine derivatives are assumed to interact with viral DNA synthesis. These three classes of compounds will be addressed in more detail, as they have been the subject of our own investigations. In addition, the potential of glycosylation inhibitors as anti-HIV agents will be briefly discussed.

Sulphated polysaccharides

Sulphated polysaccharides have proven to be very potent and selective inhibitors of HIV replication in T4 lymphocyte cultures (Ito *et al.*, 1987; Nakashima *et al.*, 1987; Ueno & Kuno, 1987; Baba *et al.*, 1988*a*, *b*). Representative congeners of this class of compounds are heparin, dextran sulphate and pentosan polysulphate (Figure 1). These compounds protect MT-4 cells against the cytopathogenicity of HIV at a concentration of 0·1-1 mg/l, while not being toxic for uninfected host cells at a concentration of 2500 mg/l, thus achieving an in-vitro therapeutic ratio (selectivity index) of approximately 10,000 (Table I).

A major liability of sulphated polysaccharides is their anticoagulant activity, which amounts to 177 U/mg for heparin. If expressed in terms of anticoagulant units, the 50% effective doses (ED_{50}) for inhibition of HIV cytopathogenicity are as follows: heparin, 0·1 U/ml; dextran sulphate, 0·0044 U/ml; pentosan polysulphate, 0·0027 U/ml. This means that the sulphated polysaccharides are inhibitory to HIV at a concentration which is ten-fold (heparin) or more than 100-fold (dextran sulphate, pentosan polysulphate) below their anticoagulant threshold (1 U).

The sulphate groups of the sulphated polysaccharides are essential for anti-HIV activity, since dextran that is lacking such sulphate groups is inactive. Likewise,

Table I. Potency and selectivity of sulphated polysaccharides against HIV in MT-4 cells

Compound	ED_{50}[a] (mg/l)	CD_{50}[b] (mg/l)	Selectivity index[c]
Heparin (MW: 11000)	0·58	>2500	> 4300
Dextran sulphate (MW: 5000)	0·3	>2500	> 8300
Pentosan polysulphate (MW: 3100)	0·19	>2500	>13150
λ-carrageenan	0·54	> 625	> 1150
Chondroitin sulphate	230	>2500	> 10
Dermatan sulphate	>625	>2500	> < 4

[a]50% effective dose, or dose required to achieve 50% protection of the cells against the cytopathic effect of HIV (based on cell viability).
[b]50% cytotoxic dose, or dose required to reduce the number of viable uninfected cells by 50%.
[c]Ratio of CD_{50} to ED_{50}.
Data taken from Baba *et al.* (1988*a*).

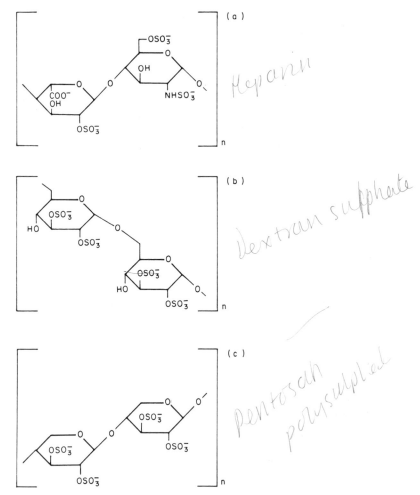

Figure 1. Repeating disaccharide units in heparin, dextran sulphate and pentosan polysulphate. Heparin (a) consists of repeating L-iduronic acid (or D-glucuronic acid)-D-glucosamine units, with sulphamides at position 2 of D-glucosamine and sulphate esters at position 6 of D-glucosamine and position 2 of L-iduronic acid (MW: 6000–20,000). Dextran sulphate (b) contains a backbone of D-glucose units linked predominantly α-D (1→6), with at an average two (or maximally three) sulphate groups per glucose unit (MW: varying from 1000 to 500,000). Pentosan polysulphate (c) can be considered as an oligomer (MW: 3100) of xylopyranose with at an average 1·8 sulphate groups per monomer.

dermatan sulphate and *N*-desulphated heparin are inactive against HIV, apparently because they do not contain a sufficient number of sulphate groups (only one per sugar unit). To achieve optimal anti-HIV activity, two to three sulphate groups per sugar unit seem required.

The importance of the molecular weight has also been assessed. For a series of dextran sulphates varying in molecular weight from 5000 to 500,000, anti-HIV activity (on a weight basis) remained remarkably constant (ED_{50}: 0·3–0·6 mg/l), which means that on a molar basis anti-HIV activity increased with increasing molecular weight (from 5000 to 500,000). Dextran sulphate with a molecular weight of 1000 was still active against HIV, although less so than the 5000-MW sample (ED_{50}: 2·8 and 0·44 mg/l, respectively when run in parallel under the same conditions).

The sulphated polysaccharides are inhibitory to the HIV-associated reverse transcriptase, but only at concentrations that are far in excess of those that inhibit viral replication in cell culture. It is unlikely therefore that an inhibitory effect on the reverse transcriptase would account for the anti-HIV activity of the sulphated polysaccharides. Instead, their anti-HIV activity could be readily attributed to an inhibitory effect on virus adsorption (Baba *et al.*, 1988*a,b*). For heparin and dextran sulphate to accomplish full anti-HIV activity, it suffices that they are present during the 2-h virus adsorption period. This results in a complete block of HIV association with the cells, as has been measured in MT-4 cell cultures exposed to radiolabelled HIV particles (Figure 2).

Dideoxynucleoside analogues

Following the initial observations of Mitsuya *et al.* (1985) and Mitsuya & Broder (1986) that 3′-azido-2′,3′-dideoxythymidine (AzddThd) and 2′,3′-dideoxynucleosides (ddCyd, ddAdo, ddIno, ddGuo and ddThd) inhibit the infectivity and cytopathic effect of HIV *in vitro*, a wide variety of 2′,3′-dideoxynucleoside analogues were found to exert a potent and selective inhibitory effect on the replication of HIV in cell culture: e.g. ddeCyd (Balzarini *et al.*, 1986, 1987*a*; Lin *et al.*, 1987*a*); ddeThd (Baba *et al.*, 1987*b*; Lin, Schinazi & Prusoff, 1987*b*; Hamamoto *et al.*, 1987); ddFCyd (Kim

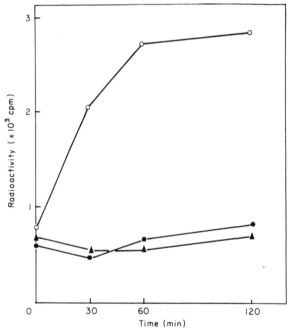

Figure 2. Effect of dextran sulphate and heparin on the adsorption of [^{32}P]orthophosphate-labelled HIV particles to MT-4 cells. The cells were incubated with the virus particles in the presence of the test compounds (25 mg/l) at 37°C for varying times (0, 30, 60 or 120 min), upon which the cells were washed and analysed for cell-associated acid-insoluble radioactivity. Data taken from Baba *et al.* (1988*b*). ○, Control; ●, dextran sulphate (25 mg/l); ▲, heparin (25 mg/l).

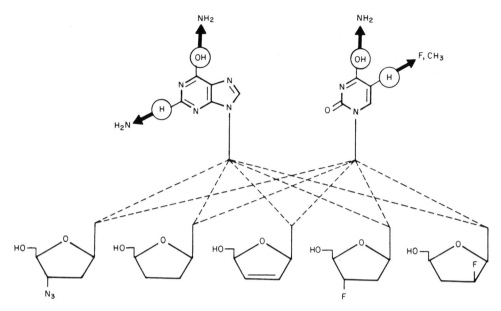

Figure 3. Unifying scheme for purine and pyrimidine 2′,3′-dideoxynucleoside analogues that have been synthesized and found active against HIV. The purine moiety may be either adenine, guanine, hypoxanthine or 2-aminoadenine (2,6-diaminopurine). The pyrimidine moiety may be either thymine, uracil, cytosine or 5-fluorocytosine. The sugar moiety may be either 2,3-dideoxyribose, 2,3-didehydro-2,3-dideoxyribose, 3-azido-2,3-dideoxyribose, 3-fluoro-2,3-dideoxyribose or 2-fluoro-2,3-dideoxyarabinose.

AzddThd:	3′-azido-2′,3′-dideoxythymidine, azidothymidine, zidovudine.
ddCyd:	2′,3′-dideoxycytidine, DDC.
ddThd:	2′,3′-dideoxythymidine.
ddeCyd:	2′,3′-didehydro-2′,3′-dideoxycytidine, D4C, dideoxycytidinene.
ddeThd:	2′,3′-didehydro-2′,3-dideoxythymidine, D4T, dideoxythymidinene.
FddCyd:	3′-fluoro-2′,3′-dideoxycytidine.
FddThd:	3′-fluoro-2′,3′-dideoxythymidine.
AzddUrd:	3′-azido-2′,3′-dideoxyuridine.
FddUrd:	3′-fluoro-2′,3′-dideoxyuridine.
ddAdo:	2′,3′-dideoxyadenosine, DDA.
AzddAdo:	3′-azido-2′,3′-dideoxyadenosine.
FddAraA:	2′-fluoro-2′,3′-dideoxy*ara*adenosine.
ddGuo:	2′,3′-dideoxyguanosine.
AzddGuo:	3′-azido-2′,3′-dideoxyguanosine.
FddGuo:	3′-fluoro-2′,3′-dideoxyguanosine.
ddDAPR:	2′,3′-dideoxy-2,6-diaminopurineriboside.
AzddDAPR:	3′-azido-2′,3′-dideoxy-2,6-diaminopurineriboside.
FddDAPR:	3′-fluoro-2′,3′-dideoxy-2,6-diaminopurineriboside.

et al., 1987); FddThd, AzddUrd, FddUrd (Herdewijn *et al.*, 1987*a*; Balzarini *et al.*, 1988*a*) and various 3′-azido-substituted pyrimidine 2′3′-dideoxyribosides (Lin *et al.*, 1988); ddDAPR (Balzarini *et al.*, 1987*b*); AzddDAPR, FddDAPR, FddGuo (Balzarini *et al.*, 1988*b*); AzddGuo (Baba *et al.*, 1987*a*); and FddAraA (Herdewijn *et al.*, 1987*b*; Marquez *et al.*, 1987). A unifying scheme for the structures of these 2′,3′-dideoxynucleoside analogues is presented in Figure 3.

From a comparative evaluation of the anti-HIV activity of these compounds (Table II), it is evident that in addition to AzddThd (zidovudine), the only drug now licensed for clinical use in the treatment of AIDS, and ddCyd (DDC) and ddAdo, the only two other drugs which are currently being examined in clinical trials, several other

Table II. Potency and selectivity of 2',3'-dideoxynucleoside analogues against HIV in MT-4 cells

Compound	$ED_{50}{}^a$ (μM)	$CD_{50}{}^b$ (μM)	Selectivity index[c]
AzddThd (zidovudine)	0·006	3·5	583
	0·004	20	5000
ddCyd (DDC)	0·06	37	616
	0·046	9·1	128
ddThd	0·2	>125	>625
ddeCyd (D4C)	0·13	7·9	61
ddeThd (D4T)	0·01	1·2	120
FddCyd	16	26	1·6
FddThd	0·001	0·197	197
AzddUrd	0·36	244	677
FddUrd	0·04	16	400
ddAdo (DDA)	6·4	890	139
AzddAdo	5	10	2
FddAraA	35	>625	>18
ddGuo	7·6	486	64
AzddGuo	1·4	190	136
FddGuo	2·4	231	96
ddDAPR	3·6	404	112
AzddDAPR	0·3	44	147
FddDAPR	4·5	360	80

[a,b,c]See footnotes to Table I.

Data taken from Baba *et al.* (1987*a,b*); Balzarini *et al.* (1987*b*, 1988*a,b*); Herdewijn *et al.* 1987*b*); Pauwels *et al.* (1987).

dideoxynucleoside analogues show a selectivity index comparable to those of zidovudine, DDC and DDA. Thus, ddThd, ddeCyd, ddeThd, FddThd, AzddUrd, FddUrd, ddGuo, AzddGuo, FddGuo, ddDAPR, AzddDAPR and FddDAPR are sufficiently potent and/or selective as anti-HIV agents to merit further investigations as potential anti-AIDS drugs. Some of these derivatives might have advantages over zidovudine, DDC or DDA from a pharmacological, pharmacokinetic or toxicological viewpoint (i.e. anti-HIV activity in a broader range of host cells, better oral absorption and/or blood-brain barrier penetration, and fewer or less severe toxic side effects). Hence these aspects should be studied with as many of the new congeners as possible.

The mechanism of action of all dideoxynucleoside analogues may be quite similar to that of zidovudine involving successive phosphorylation to their 5'-mono-, 5'-di- and 5'-triphosphate derivatives by cellular enzymes, followed by a specific interaction of the latter with the HIV reverse transcriptase (Figure 4). Cellular DNA polymerases α and β are much less sensitive to inhibition by zidovudine 5'-triphosphate than the viral reverse transcriptase (Furman *et al.*, 1986; St Clair *et al.*, 1987), which points to the reverse transcriptase as a specific target for antiviral chemotherapy. Other 2',3'-dideoxynucleoside 5'-triphosphates (ddNTPs) have also been examined for their inhibitory effects on HIV reverse transcriptase (Ono *et al.*, 1986; Vrang *et al.*, 1987; Cheng *et al.*, 1987; Matthes *et al.*, 1987; Chen & Oshana, 1987); and ddeTTP, ddTTP and FddTTP proved at least as inhibitory, if not more inhibitory, to HIV reverse transcriptase than AzddTTP (Cheng *et al.*, 1987; Matthes *et al.*, 1987).

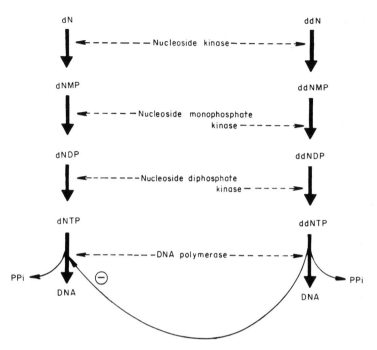

Figure 4. Mechanism of action of 2′,3′-dideoxynucleoside (ddN) analogues. Akin to their 2′-deoxynucleoside counterparts (dN), the 2′,3′-dideoxynucleosides are successively converted to the 5′-monophosphates (dNMP, ddNMP), 5′-diphosphates (dNDP, ddNDP) and 5′-triphosphates (dNTP, ddNTP). The ddNTPs then interfere with the DNA polymerase, having, as a rule, a greater affinity for the HIV-associated reverse transcriptase than for cellular DNA polymerases. The ddNTPs can serve as either inhibitors or substrates of the DNA polymerase reaction. As inhibitors they act competitively with respect to the natural substrates (dNTPs). When functioning themselves as substrates for the enzyme, they are incorporated at the 3′-terminal and prevent further chain elongation.

Phosphonylmethoxyethyl purine derivatives

Recently we identified a new class of acyclic nucleotide analogues (Figure 5) as potent and selective inhibitors of HIV. The prototype of this class, (S)-9-(3-hydroxy-2-phosphonylmethoxypropyl)adenine ((S)-HPMPA) has a broad antiviral activity spectrum, encompassing all major herpes viruses as well as adeno-, pox- and iridoviruses (De Clercq *et al.*, 1986, 1987). The structurally related compound 9-(2-phosphonylmethoxyethyl)adenine (PMEA) is equally active as (S)-HPMPA against herpes simplex virus (HSV) but significantly less active against varicella-zoster virus, cytomegalovirus, adenovirus and vaccinia virus. On the other hand, PMEA is particularly active against retroviruses, i.e. murine (Moloney) sarcoma virus (MSV) and HIV, and so are the closely related congeners of PMEA, PMEMAP and PMEDAP (Table III) (Pauwels *et al.*, 1988). The anti-retrovirus activity of PMEA also extends to the in-vivo situation, where it was found to be significantly more potent and also more selective than zidovudine in suppressing MSV-induced tumour development, and associated mortality, in newborn mice (Balzarini, J., Naesens, L., Herdewijn, P., Rosenberg, I., Holy, A., Pauwels, R. *et al.*, unpublished observations).

The mechanism of action of PMEA remains to be elucidated. For its closely related congener, (S)-HPMPA, it has been ascertained that the compound can as such be taken up by the cells. It is subsequently converted to its mono- and diphosphoryl

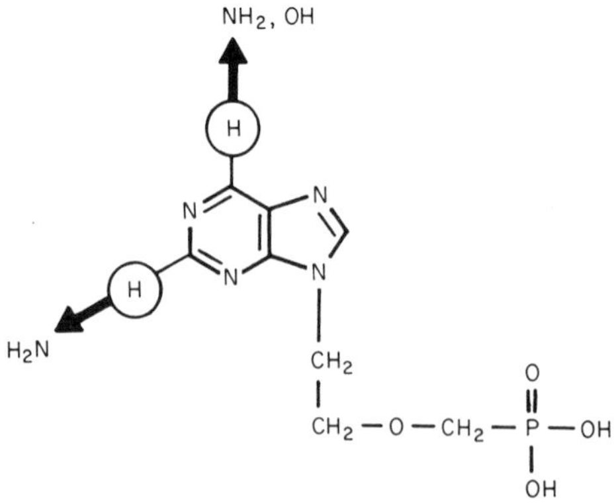

Figure 5. 9-(2-Phosphonylmethoxyethyl)purine derivatives that have been synthesized and evaluated for anti-HIV activity.

PMEA: 9-(2-phosphonylmethoxyethyl)adenine.
PMEMAP: 9-(2-phosphonylmethoxyethyl)-2-monoaminopurine.
PMEDAP: 9-(2-phosphonylmethoxyethyl)-2,6-diaminopurine.
PMEG: 9-(2-phosphonylmethoxyethyl)guanine.
PMEHx: 9-(2-phosphonylmethoxyethyl)hypoxanthine.

derivative by cellular enzymes. The latter may well be the active form of the molecule. (S)-HPMPA inhibits viral DNA synthesis at concentrations which are by several orders of magnitude lower than those required for inhibition of cellular DNA synthesis. This has been demonstrated with both HSV- and Epstein-Barr virus (EBV)-infected cells (Votruba *et al.*, 1987; Lin, De Clercq & Pagano, 1987). In fact PMEA also effects a specific inhibition of EBV DNA synthesis (Lin *et al.*, 1987), and, likewise, its anti-HIV activity may be attributed to a specific inhibition of the viral RNA-directed DNA synthesis.

Glycosylation inhibitors

Since the viral envelope gp 120 glycoprotein involved in the binding of HIV to the CD4 receptor is heavily glycosylated (31–36 N-linked glycans per gp 120 molecule), glycosylation inhibitors have been considered as a potential means to inhibit HIV infectivity and, hence, suppress spread of the virus. The first glycosylation inhibitor shown to inhibit the expression of HIV envelope glycoproteins was 2-deoxy-D-glucose

Table III. Potency and selectivity of 9-(2-phosphonylmethoxy-ethyl)purine derivatives against HIV in MT-4 cells

Compound	ED_{50}[a] (μM)	CD_{50}[b] (μM)	Selectivity index[c]
PMEA	2·0	67	33·5
PMEMAP	45	1250	>28
PMEDAP	1·0	18	18
PMEG	3·8	11	3
PMEHx	>125	>625	><5

[a,b,c]See footnotes to Table I.
Data taken from Pauwels *et al.* (1988).

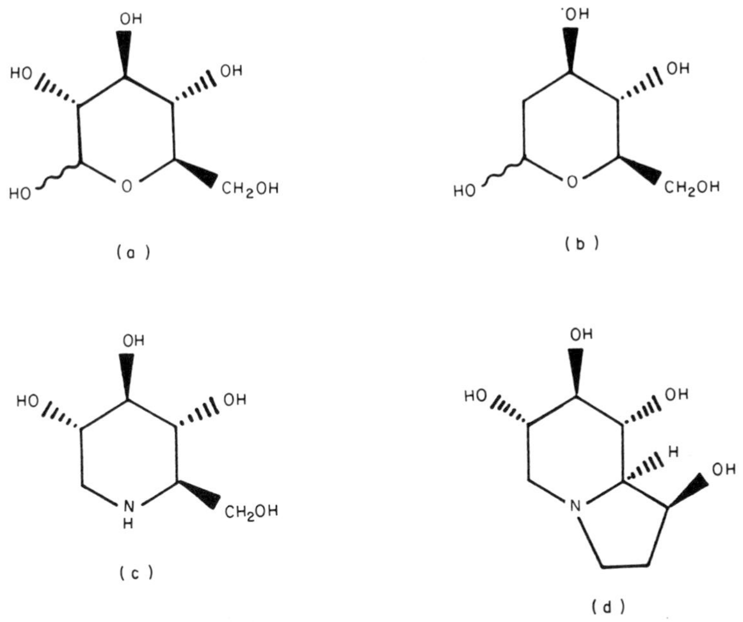

Figure 6. Glycosylation inhibitors: 2-deoxyglucose, 1-deoxynojirimycin and castanospermine. The latter (1,6,7,8-tetrahydroxyoctahydroindolizine) is a plant alkaloid isolated from seeds of the Australian chestnut tree *Castanospermum australe*. Castanospermine and 1-deoxynojirimycin inhibit the glucosidases that are responsible for the removal of glucose residues during the trimming process of the glycoproteins. This trimming is necessary for the 'core' oligosaccharides to be converted to the 'terminal' oligosaccharides. Castanospermine and 1-deoxynojirimycin are inhibitors of HIV infection. A related glycosylation inhibitor, 1-deoxymannojirimycin, which interferes with the mannosidases involved in the trimming process does not inhibit HIV infection (Gruters *et al.*, 1987). (a) Glucose; (b) 2-deoxyglucose; (c) 1-deoxynojirimycin; (d) castanospermine.

(Figure 6) (Blough *et al.*, 1986). 2-Deoxy-glucose only did so at a very high concentration (5 mM).

More recently, other glycosylation inhibitors such as castanospermine and 1-deoxynojirimycin (Figure 6) have been found to inhibit HIV infectivity and HIV-induced syncytium formation (Gruters *et al.*, 1987; Tyms *et al.*, 1987; Walker *et al.*, 1987). The decrease in syncytium formation in the presence of castanospermine can be attributed to inhibition of cell surface expression of the mature gp 120 (Walker *et al.*, 1987). Both castanospermine and 1-deoxynojirimycin, but not the closely related 1-deoxymannojirimycin, are active against retroviruses (Gruters *et al.*, 1987; Sunkara *et al.*, 1987). This differential behaviour may be related to differences in the mode of action of these three glycosylation inhibitors: castanospermine and 1-deoxynojirimycin inhibit the glucosidases, whereas 1-deoxymannojirimycin inhibits the mannosidases involved in the trimming of the *N*-linked oligosaccharides.

Glycosylation inhibitors obviously deserve further attention as potential anti-HIV agents. Castanospermine and 1-deoxynojirimycin inhibit the replication of HIV at concentrations (i.e., 1 mM, according to our own experience and that of Gruters *et al.* (1987)) which do not affect the growth of uninfected host cells. It is questionable, however, whether such high concentrations could ever be attained *in vivo*. Also, it is not known whether castanospermine, or any other glycosylation inhibitor, has therapeutic efficacy against retrovirus infections in animal models.

When designing new glycosylation inhibitors, it may be worthwhile to envisage one of the final steps in the glycosylation process, i.e. the addition of N-acetylneuraminic acid (NANA), as this may be one of the targets where the greatest specificity could be achieved.

Acknowledgements

The author is indebted to all his coworkers, and in particular J. Balzarini, M. Baba, P. Herdewijn, R. Pauwels and D. Schols, who participated in the original investigations. These investigations were supported by grants from the Belgian Fonds voor Geneeskundig Wetenschappelijk Onderzoek (Projects no. 3.0040.83 and no. 3.0097.87) and the Belgian Geconcerteerde Onderzoeksacties (Project no. 85/90-79), by the AIDS Basic Research Programme of the European Community and by Janssen Pharmaceutica. The excellent editorial help of Christiane Callebaut is gratefully acknowledged.

References

Baba, M., Pauwels, R., Balzarini, J., Herdewijn, P. & De Clercq, E. (1987a). Selective inhibition of human immunodeficiency virus (HIV) by 3'-azido-2',3'-dideoxyguanosine *in vitro*. *Biochemical and Biophysical Research Communications* **145**, 1080–6.

Baba, M., Pauwels, R., Herdewijn, P., De Clercq, E., Desmyter, J. & Vandeputte, M. (1987b). Both 2',3'-dideoxythymidine and its 2',3'-unsaturated derivative (2',3'-dideoxythymidinene) are potent and selective inhibitors of human immunodeficiency virus replication in vitro. *Biochemical and Biophysical Research Communications* **142**, 128–34.

Baba, M., Nakajima, M., Schols, D., Pauwels, R., Balzarini, J. & De Clercq, E. (1988a). Pentosan polysulfate, a sulfated oligosaccharide, is a potent and selective anti-HIV agent in vitro *Antiviral Research*, in press.

Baba, M., Pauwels, R., Balzarini, J., Arnout, J., Desmyter, J. & De Clercq, E. (1988b). Mechanism of inhibitory effect of dextran sulfate and heparin on the replication of human immunodeficiency virus *in vitro*. *Proceedings of the National Academy of Sciences of the United States of America*, in press.

Balzarini, J., Pauwels, R., Herdewijn, P., De Clercq, E., Cooney, D. A., Kang, G.-J. *et al.* (1986). Potent and selective anti-HTLV-III/LAV activity of 2',3'-dideoxycytidinene, the 2',3'-unsaturated derivative of 2',3'-dideoxycytidine. *Biochemical and Biophysical Research Communications* **140**, 735–42.

Balzarini, J., Kang, G.-J., Dalal, M., Herdewijn, P., De Clercq, E., Broder, S. *et al.* (1987a). The anti-HTLV-III (anti-HIV) and cytotoxic activity of 2',3'-didehydro-2',3'-dideoxy-ribonucleosides: a comparison with their parental 2',3'-dideoxyribonucleosides. *Molecular Pharmacology* **32**, 162–7.

Balzarini, J., Pauwels, R., Baba, M., Robins, M. J., Zou, R., Herdewijn, P., *et al.* (1987b). The 2',3'-dideoxyriboside of 2,6-diaminopurine selectively inhibits human immunodeficiency virus (HIV) replication *in vitro*. *Biochemical and Biophysical Research Communications* **145**, 269–76.

Balzarini, J., Baba, M., Pauwels, R., Herdewijn, P. & De Clercq, E. (1988a). Anti-retrovirus activity of 3'-fluoro- and 3'-azido-substituted pyrimidine 2',3'-dideoxynucleoside analogues. *Biochemical Pharmacology*, in press.

Balzarini, J., Baba, M., Pauwels, R., Herdewijn, P., Wood, S. G., Robins, M. J., *et al.* (1988b). Potent and selective activity of 3'-azido-2,6-diaminopurine-2',3'-dideoxyriboside, 3'-fluoro-2,6-diaminopurine-2',3'-dideoxyriboside, and 3'-fluoro-2',3'-dideoxyguanosine against human immunodeficiency virus. *Molecular Pharmacology* **33**, 243–9.

Blough, H. A., Pauwels, R., De Clercq, E., Cogniaux, J., Sprecher-Goldberger, S. & Thiry, L. (1986). Glycosylation inhibitors block the expression of LAV/HTLV-III (HIV) glycoproteins. *Biochemical and Biophysical Research Communications* **141**, 33–8.

Chen, M. S. & Oshana, S. C. (1987). Inhibition of HIV reverse transcriptase by 2′,3′-dideoxynucleoside triphosphates. *Biochemical Pharmacology* **36**, 4361–2.

Cheng, Y.-C., Dutschman, G. E., Bastow, K. F., Sarngadharan, M. G. & Ting, R. Y. C. (1987). Human immunodeficiency virus reverse transcriptase. *Journal of Biological Chemistry* **262**, 2187–9.

De Clercq, E., Holý, A., Rosenberg, I., Sakuma, T., Balzarini, J. & Maudgal, P. C. (1986). A novel selective broad-spectrum anti-DNA virus agent. *Nature* **323**, 464–7.

De Clercq, E., Sakuma, T., Baba, M., Pauwels, R., Balzarini, J., Rosenberg, I., *et al.* (1987). Antiviral activity of phosphonylmethoxyalkyl derivatives of purine and pyrimidines. *Antiviral Research* **8**, 261–72.

Furman, P. A., Fyfe, J. A., St. Clair, M. H., Weinhold, K., Rideout, J. L., Freeman, G. A., *et al.* (1986). Phosphorylation of 3′-azido-3′-deoxythymidine and selective interaction of the 5′-triphosphate with human immunodeficiency virus reverse transcriptase. *Proceedings of the National Academy of Sciences of the United States of America* **83**, 8333–7.

Gruters, R. A., Neefjes, J. J., Tersmette, M., de Goede, R. E. Y., Tulp, A., Huisman, H. G., *et al.* (1987). Interference with HIV-induced syncytium formation and viral infectivity by inhibitors of trimming glucosidase. *Nature* **330**, 74–7.

Hamamoto, Y., Nakashima, H., Matsui, T., Matsuda, A., Ueda, T. & Yamamoto, N. (1987). Inhibitory effect of 2′,3′-didehydro-2′,3′-dideoxynucleosides on infectivity, cytopathic effects, and replication of human immunodeficiency virus. *Antimicrobial Agents and Chemotherapy* **31**, 907–10.

Herdewijn, P., Balzarini, J., De Clercq, E., Pauwels, R., Baba, M., Broder, S., *et al.* (1987*a*). 3′-Substituted 2′,3′-dideoxynucleoside analogues as potential anti-HIV (HTLV-III/LAV) agents. *Journal of Medicinal Chemistry* **30**, 1270–8.

Herdewijn, P., Pauwels, R., Baba, M., Balzarini, J. & De Clercq, E. (1987*b*). Synthesis and anti-HIV activity of various 2′- and 3′-substituted 2′,3′-dideoxyadenosines: a structure-activity analysis. *Journal of Medicinal Chemistry* **30**, 2131–7.

Ito, M., Baba, M., Sato, A., Pauwels, R., De Clercq, E. & Shigeta, S. (1987). Inhibitory effect of dextran sulfate and heparin on the replication of human immunodeficiency virus (HIV) in vitro. *Antiviral Research* **7**, 361–7.

Kim, C.-H., Marquez, V. E., Broder, S., Mitsuya, H. & Driscoll, J. S. (1987). Potential anti-AIDS drugs. 2′,3′-Dideoxycytidine analogues. *Journal of Medicinal Chemistry* **30**, 862–6.

Lin, J.-C., De Clercq, E. & Pagano, J. S. (1987). Novel acyclic adenosine analogs inhibit Epstein-Barr virus replication. *Antimicrobial Agents and Chemotherapy* **31**, 1431–3.

Lin, T.-S., Guo, J.-Y., Schinazi, R. F., Chu, C. K., Xiang, J.-N. & Prusoff, W. H. (1988). Synthesis and antiviral activity of various 3′-azido analogues of pyrimidine deoxy-ribonucleosides against human immunodeficiency virus (HIV-1, HTLV-III/LAV). *Journal of Medicinal Chemistry* **31**, 336–40.

Lin, T.-S., Schinazi, R. F., Chen, M. S., Kinney-Thomas, E. & Prusoff, W. H. (1987*a*). Antiviral activity of 2′,3′-dideoxycytidin-2′-ene (2′,3′-dideoxy-2′,3′-didehydrocytidine) against human immunodeficiency virus *in vitro*. *Biochemical Pharmacology* **36**, 311–6.

Lin, T.-S., Schinazi, R. F. & Prusoff, W. H. (1987*b*). Potent and selective *in vitro* activity of 3′-deoxythymidin-2′-ene (3′-deoxy-2′,3′-didehydrothymidine) against human immuno-deficiency virus. *Biochemical Pharmacology* **36**, 2713–8.

Marquez, V. E., Tseng, C. K.-H., Kelley, J. A., Mitsuya, H., Broder, S., Roth, J. S., *et al.* (1987). 2′,3′-Dideoxy-2′-fluoro-ara-A. An acid-stable purine nucleoside active against human immunodeficiency virus (HIV). *Biochemical Pharmacology* **36**, 2719–22.

Matthes, E., Lehmann, Ch., Scholz, D., von Janta-Lipinski, M., Gaertner, K., Rosenthal, H. A., *et al.* (1987). Inhibition of HIV-associated reverse transcriptase by sugar-modified derivatives of thymidine 5′-triphosphate in comparison to cellular DNA polymerases α and β. *Biochemical and Biophysical Research Communications* **148**, 78–85.

Mitsuya, H. & Broder, S. (1986). Inhibition of the *in vitro* infectivity and cytopathic effect of human T-lymphotrophic virus type III/lymphadenopathy-associated virus (HTLV-III/LAV) by 2′,3′-dideoxynucleosides. *Proceedings of the National Academy of Sciences of the United States of America* **83**, 911–5.

Mitsuya, H., Weinhold, K. J., Furman, P. A., St. Clair, M. H., Nusinoff Lehrman, S., Gallo, R. C., *et al.* (1985). 3′-Azido-3′-deoxythymidine (BW A509U): an antiviral agent that inhibits the infectivity and cytopathic effect of human T-lymphotropic virus type III/lymphadeno-pathy-associated virus *in vitro. Proceedings of the National Academy of Sciences of the United States of America* **82**, 7096–100.

Nakashima, H., Kido, Y., Kobayashi, N., Motoki, Y., Neushul, M. & Yamamoto, N. (1987). Purification and characterization of an avian myeloblastosis and human immunodeficiency virus reverse transcriptase inhibitor, sulfated polysaccharides extracted from sea algae. *Antimicrobial Agents and Chemotherapy* **31**, 1524–8.

Ono, K., Ogasawara, M., Iwata, Y., Nakane, H., Fujii, T., Sawai, K., *et al.* (1986). Inhibition of reverse transcriptase activity by 2′,3′-dideoxythymidine 5′-triphosphate and its derivatives modified on the 3′ position. *Biochemical and Biophysical Research Communications* **140**, 498–507.

Pauwels, R., De Clercq, E., Desmyter, J., Balzarini, J., Goubau, P., Herdewijn, P., *et al.* (1987). Sensitive and rapid assay on MT-4 cells for detection of antiviral compounds against the AIDS virus. *Journal of Virological Methods* **16**, 171–85.

Pauwels, R., Balzarini, J., Schols, D., Baba, M., Desmyter, J., Rosenberg, I., *et al.* (1988). Phosphonylmethoxyethyl purine derivatives: a new class of anti-HIV agents. *Antimicrobial Agents and Chemotherapy,* in press.

St. Clair, M. H., Richards, C. A., Spector, T., Weinhold, K. J., Miller, W. H., Langlois, A. J., *et al.* (1987). 3′-Azido-3′-deoxythymidine triphosphate as an inhibitor and substrate of purified human immunodeficiency virus reverse transcriptase. *Antimicrobial Agents and Chemotherapy* **31**, 1972–7.

Sunkara, P. S., Bowlin, T. L., Liu, P. S. & Sjoerdsma, A. (1987). Antiretroviral activity of castanospermine and deoxynojirimycin, specific inhibitors of glycoprotein processing. *Biochemical and Biophysical Research Communications* **148**, 206–10.

Traunecker, A., Lüke, W. & Karjalainen, K. (1988). Soluble CD4 molecules neutralize human immunodeficiency virus type 1. *Nature* **331**, 84–6.

Tyms, A. S., Berrie, E. M., Ryder, T. A., Nash, R. J., Hegarty, M. P., Taylor, D. L., Mobberley, M. A., *et al.* (1987). Castanospermine and other plant alkaloid inhibitors of glucosidase activity block the growth of HIV. *Lancet* **ii**, 1025–6.

Ueno, R. & Kuno, S. (1987). Dextran sulphate, a potent anti-HIV agent in vitro having synergism with zidovudine. *Lancet* **i**, 1379.

Votruba, I., Bernaerts, R., Sakuma, T., De Clercq, E., Merta, A., Rosenberg, I., *et al.* (1987). Intracellular phosphorylation of broad-spectrum anti-DNA virus agent (S)-9-(3-hydroxy-2-phosphonylmethoxypropyl)adenine and inhibition of viral DNA synthesis. *Molecular Pharmacology* **32**, 524–9.

Vrang, L., Bazin, H., Remaud, G., Chattopadhyaya, J. & Öberg, B. (1987). Inhibition of the reverse transcriptase from HIV by 3′-azido-3′-deoxythymidine triphosphate and its *threo* analogue. *Antiviral Research* **7**, 139–49.

Walker, B. D., Kowalski, M., W. C., Kozarsky, K., Krieger, M., Rosen, C., *et al.* (1987). Inhibition of human immunodeficiency virus syncytium formation and virus replication by castanospermine. *Proceedings of the National Academy of Sciences of the United States of America* **84**, 8120–4.

Journal of Antimicrobial Chemotherapy (1989) **23**, Suppl. A, 47–54

Structural characterization of HIV reverse transcriptase: a target for the design of specific virus inhibitors

M. Tisdale, B. A. Larder, D. M. Lowe, D. K. Stammers, D. J. M. Purifoy, P. Ertl, C. Bradley, S. Kemp, G. K. Darby and K. L. Powell

Department of Molecular Sciences, Wellcome Research Laboratories, Langley Court, Beckenham, Kent BR3 3BS, UK

The reverse transcriptase (RT) of HIV is an important target for chemotherapy as demonstrated by the effective treatment of AIDS patients with zidovudine, a potent inhibitor of RT. Structural studies of HIV RT were therefore undertaken with a view to designing more effective inhibitors. To obtain sufficient quantities of enzyme for these studies the reverse transcriptase gene of HIV was cloned into a high level expression plasmid yielding reverse transcriptase at a level of 10% of the total *Escherichia coli* proteins. Monoclonal antibodies to RT were raised in mice and have been used to purify the enzyme by immunoaffinity chromatography. Crystallization of the enzyme has been achieved and studies are underway to determine its three-dimensional structure. In addition, carboxy-terminal truncated mutants were prepared by inserting stop codons into the gene at appropriate sites. The proteins expressed were analysed for RT and RNase H activity and used for mapping RT epitopes. This, together with previous data on site-directed mutagenesis of conserved regions of HIV RT has helped to map some of the structural and functional regions of the enzyme.

Introduction

The development of inhibitors of HIV is one of the major goals in the fight to control the AIDS epidemic. As a result of large scale screening programmes several inhibitors of HIV replication in tissue culture have been identified, including some nucleoside analogues (De Clercq & Balzarini, 1985; Mitsuya & Broder, 1987). One nucleoside analogue, zidovudine, has been shown to give significant clinical benefit to AIDS patients, reducing HIV-Ag levels in serum. (Chaisson *et al.*, 1986; Fischl *et al.*, 1987). Zidovudine is phosphorylated by cellular enzymes to the 5' triphosphate which has been shown to be a potent inhibitor of HIV reverse transcriptase (Furman *et al.*, 1986). Reverse transcriptase (RT) is an essential enzyme in retrovirus replication which converts viral RNA into a double stranded DNA copy before integration into the host cell genome (Weiss *et al.*, 1985). The clinical success of zidovudine has established that HIV RT is a good target for the development of anti-HIV drugs. An alternative approach to that of screening compounds against HIV in tissue culture involves the design of inhibitors to specifically fit the active site of one of the virus enzymes based on its 3-D structure. We have chosen to apply this approach to the study of HIV RT.

The enzyme has been shown, using monoclonal antibodies, to be present in the virus, as two polypeptides of 66 and 51 kd molecular weight (di Marzo Veronese *et al.*,

1986; Tisdale *et al.*, 1988) (Figure 1). These two polypeptides share a common amino terminus (di Marzo Veronese *et al.*, 1986) and the 51 kd polypeptide appears to be derived from the 66 kd polypeptide by cleavage of approximately 130 amino acids from the C-terminus (Hansen *et al.*, 1988; Tisdale *et al.*, 1988). From comparative amino acid sequence analysis of several retrovirus *pol* genes plus *Escherichia coli* DNA-directed RNA polymerase and RNase H genes, Johnson *et al.* (1986) constructed a map for the RT gene with functional homology to reverse transcriptases within the N-terminal half of the molecule and functional homology to RNase H near the C-terminus, with a structural 'tether' region separating these two regions. We have taken these studies further and identified six regions within the N-terminal half of the molecule with high homology within reverse transcriptases and one region possessing homology also with RNA polymerases (Larder *et al.*, 1987*a*). In addition, Hansen *et*

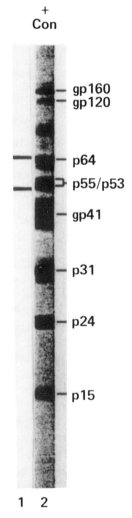

+
Con

— gp160
— gp120

— p64
— p55/p53
— gp41
— p31
— p24
— p15

1   2

Figure 1. Detection of RT related polypeptides in preparations of HIV particles (Dupont Western Blot Kit) using monoclonal antibody RTMAb6 (panel 1) in comparison with a human AIDS patient serum (panel 2).

al. (1988) have demonstrated that the 66 kd viral polypeptide and a 15 kd polypeptide derived from the C-terminus possess RNase H activity.

Although significant studies have been carried out on enzyme purified from the virus, to obtain sufficient quantities of enzyme for 3-D structural studies it was necessary to clone and express the RT in *E. coli.*

Production and purification of recombinant HIV reverse transcriptase

We obtained a sub-genomic clone of the AIDS genome (pSHGP-1) from Dr Malcolm Martin at The National Institute of Health (NIH, USA) containing the *pol* gene. The *pol* gene encodes for three proteins, a protease, reverse transcriptase and an endonuclease, which are made as a polyprotein and subsequently cleaved with virus infected cells. A BgIII-EcoRI fragment of the *pol* gene was cloned into an M13 phage system, mptac18 (Larder *et al.*, 1987*b*). A series of genetic manipulations were carried out, firstly to remove the endonuclease sequence leaving a HindIII site at the 3′ end of the RT sequence, and secondly to remove the protease sequences, creating a new EcoRI site at the 5′ end of the RT sequence. A construct was thus obtained containing just the RT gene sequence which gave high level RT activity (Figure 2) and a 66 kd polypeptide on gels. To obtain sufficient protein for crystallization studies the RT 'cassette' from mpRT4 was inserted into a high level expression plasmid pKK233-2 which on induction in *E. coli* produced the RT polypeptide at levels of about 10% of the *E. coli* total protein.

The 66 kd polypeptide was purified by a combination of DNA cellulose and anion exchange chromatography (Larder *et al.*, 1987*b*) and used to raise monoclonal antibodies in mice. Eight monoclonal antibodies were isolated which were blotted against high levels of purified bacterially expressed 66 kd RT which contained low levels of the 51 kd polypeptide. Seven of the monoclonal antibodies reacted with both

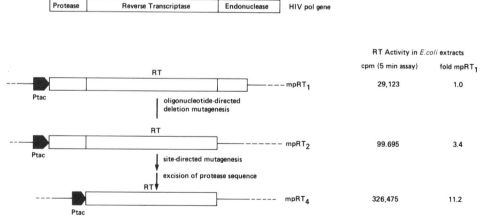

Figure 2. Cloning and expression of HIV RT activity in *E. coli*. The upper map indicates the relative positions of protease and endonuclease coding sequences to those encoding RT. The lower maps illustrate the steps in refining the RT expressing construct and the associated RT activity of each construct induced in *E. coli* with infection by phage. [Reproduced from The Embo Journal 6, 3133, (1987) with permission from IRL press].

the 66 and 51 kd polypeptides, however one, RTMAb 8, reacted with only the 66 kd polypeptide (Figure 3). Since we wished to obtain pure 66 kd polypeptide for crystallization studies, RTMAb 8 was used to prepare an immunoabsorbent column. Crude bacterial extracts were prepared by high salt fractionation and purified by immunoaffinity chromatography. Extracts of RT were applied to the column in 50 mM diethylamine buffer pH 8·8 with 0·1 M sodium chloride. After washing the column with buffer, the RT was eluted using 50% ethylene glycol in DEA buffer pH 8·8. Fractions were analysed on 7·5% polyacrylamide gels and stained with Kenacid Blue R (Figure 4). By this purification process large quantities of purified 66 kd polypeptide have been obtained. Using this material crystallization of the RT has been achieved and X-ray crystallographic studies of the pure enzyme are underway.

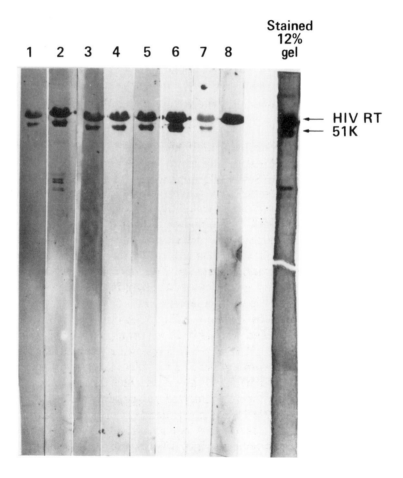

Figure 3. Western blots with RT monoclonal antibodies 1 to 8 against high levels of purified bacterially expressed 66 kd RT containing low levels of the 51kd polypeptide.

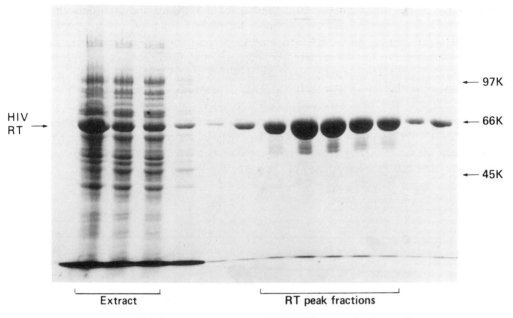

Figure 4. Purification of 66 kd RT using RTMAb8 immunoabsorbent column.

Mapping of RT antibody epitopes, RT and RNase H functional regions of the 66 kd polypeptide

Carboxy-terminal truncated mutants, prepared by introducing premature stop codons within the RT gene in the M13 construct mpRT4, were used to map the epitopes of the monoclonal antibodies and to examine both RT and RNase H activity of the mutant polypeptides produced. Epitope mapping was carried out by Western blot analysis of the different polypeptides induced in *E. coli*. *E. coli* cells were infected with the M13 constructs and induced with IPTG (15 h) and extracts were prepared and run on gels for staining and blotting. RT activity was determined in crude bacterial extracts using an *E. coli* strain ($5KCPo1A^{ts}F'$) which has a ts defect its polymerase gene, allowing accurate determination of mutant IT activity. Five microlitres of each extract was taken for assays of RT activity using Poly (rA)-oligo(dT) as primer template. For RNase H determinations, because of high levels of *E. coli* RNase H, it was necessary to purify the polypeptides by immuno-affinity chromatography. For mutant polypeptides which do not bind RTMAb 8, an immunoabsorbent column was prepared using RTMAb 3. RNase H assays were carried out using ^{3}H Poly(rA)-Poly(dT) as template with a series of time points taken over 30 mins at 37°C, and TCA soluble activity determined i.e. radioactivity released from the template.

Six constructs producing a range of truncated polypeptides were prepared to map the epitope for RTMAb 8 (Table I). These revealed that the epitope must lie close to the C-terminus within amino acids 531–539. RT and RNase H analysis indicated that the 66kD polypeptide possessed both activities, whereas the 51kD polypeptide made to mimic the 51kD polypeptide in virus possessed significant but reduced RT activity (20 × lower than the 66kD polypeptide) but no RNase H activity. The polypeptide expressed by CTRT14 which has 21 amino acids removed from the C-terminus had

Table I. C-terminus truncated mutants of RT: binding to RTMAb 8, reverse transcriptase and RNase H activity

M13 construct Structure	Name	Apparent M_r of RT polypeptide $(\times 10^3)$	Detection by Western blot with RT MAb 8	RT activity % mpRT4	RNaseH activity
N————^{560}aa————C	mpRT4	66	+	100	+
N————^{430}aa——C	CTRT1	53·5	−	5	−
N————^{531}aa————C	CTRT2	65	−	30	(−)
N————^{539}aa————C	CTRT14	65·3	+	100	(−)
N————^{543}aa————C	CTRT12	65·8	+	100	ND
N————^{549}aa————C	CTRT10	66	+	100	ND
N————^{554}aa————C	CTRT9	66·6	+	100	ND

ND, not determined; (−), only very low level activity detected which may be from *E. coli* RNase H contamination.

high level RT activity but little or no RNase H activity suggesting that this end of the molecule is important to RNase H function. The drop in RT activity seen when 28–130 amino acids are removed from the C-terminus probably arises from changes in the tertiary structure of the polypeptide.

Monoclonal antibodies 1 to 7 were mapped using a combination of cyanogen bromide fragmentation of RT and preparation of further C-terminus truncated mutants. All seven antibodies mapped to a region within amino acids 233–317 and probably lie within the region 296–317.

Taking the above results together with those from studies on site-directed mutagenesis of conserved RT functional regions and subsequent analysis of the mutant polypeptides sensitivity to zidovudine and phosphonoformic acid (PFA), it has been possible to construct a linear map of the structural and functional regions of the HIV RT polypeptide (Figure 5). These observations substantiate the map suggested by Johnson *et al.* (1986). Within the N-terminal half of the molecule mutants in two regions, B and C, (Figure 5) show decreased sensitivity to both PFA and zidovudine suggesting that these two regions are involved with pyrophosphate exchange and triphosphate binding. Whereas mutants in region F show decreased sensitivity to zidovudine only, suggesting involvement with triphosphate binding. Mutants in region E, which shares homology with RNA polymerases, have either lost or show low level RT activity. Analysis of the mutant from region E, with low level RT activity, showed no change in sensitivity to zidovudine and PFA, which supports the suggestion that this region may be involved with template binding (Kamar & Argos, 1984).

The monoclonal antibodies 1 to 7 do not neutralize RT activity indicating that they are probably binding to a non-functional region of the molecule which is consistent with the 'tether' region consisting of amino acids 269-441 (Johnson *et al.*, 1986). Finally, the results with the C-terminal truncated mutants strongly support the homology data that amino acids at the C-terminal end of the molecule are involved with RNase H function.

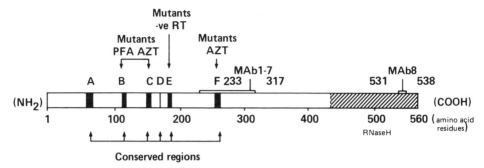

Figure 5. Linear map of the amino acid sequence of HIV RT indicating structural and functional regions of the molecule. Regions labelled A to F indicate RT functional conserved regions. Monoclonal antibody epitopes are indicated as is the region containing R Nase H function (cross-hatched). AZT, Zidovudine; PFA, phosphonoformic acid.

From these studies on mutant enzymes important functional regions of the molecule have been identified. This, together with 3-D structural information which we hope to obtain from the crystallographic studies should enable the rational design of inhibitors to RT and to RNase H function. In addition, the large quantities of enzyme obtained from *E. coli*, which behaves like authentic viral enzyme, have allowed large numbers of compounds to be tested as inhibitors of reverse transcriptase.

Similar studies on other viral gene products will not only increase our understanding of HIV replication but increase the chances of developing highly specific non-nucleoside inhibitors to this important virus. Drug discovery in the antiviral area is moving rapidly from the blind approach of screening nucleosides for activity to the specific design of new agents based on more detailed information on viral enzymes but it is to be expected that in the short term purines and pyrimidines will remain vitally important to the clinical treatment of AIDS. Drug combinations involving inhibitors to two or more viral target products may be the most successful means of controlling or even eradicating HIV from infected individuals.

References

Chaisson, R. E., Allain, J.-P., Leuther, M. & Volberding, P. A. (1986). Significant changes in HIV antigen level in the serum of patients treated with azidothymidine. *New England Journal of Medicine* **315**, 1610–1.

De Clercq, E. & Balzarini, J. (1985). In search of specific inhibitors of retrovirus replication. *Antiviral Research 5, Suppl. 1*, 89–94.

di Marzo Veronese, F., Copeland, T. D., De Vico, A. L., Rahman R. Oroszlan, S., Gallo, R. C. *et al.* (1986). Characterization of highly immunogenic p66/p51 as the reverse transcriptase of HTLV-III/LAV. *Science* **231**, 1289–91.

Fischl, M. A., Richmann, D. D., Grieco, M. H., Gottlieb, M. S., Volberding, P. A., Laskin, O. L. *et al.* (1987). The efficacy of azidothymidine (AZT) in the treatment of patients with AIDS and AIDS-related complex. *New England Journal of Medicine* **317**, 185–91.

Furman, P. A., Fyfe, J. A., St Clair, M. H., Weinhold, K., Rideout, J. L., Freeman, G. A. *et al.* (1986). Phosphorylation of 3'-azido-3'-deoxythymidine and selective interaction of the 5'-triphosphate with human immunodeficiency virus reverse transcriptase. *Proceedings of the National Academy of Sciences USA* **83**, 8333–7.

Hansen, J., Schulze, T., Mellert, W. & Moelling, K. (1988). Identification and characterization of HIV-specific RNase H by monoclonal antibody. *EMBO Journal* **7**, 239–43.

Johnson, M. S., McClure, M. A., Feng, D. F., Gray, J. & Doolittle, R. F. (1986). Computer analysis of retroviral pol genes: Assignment of enzymatic functions to specific sequences and homologies with nonviral enzymes. *Proceedings of the National Academy of Sciences USA* **83**, 7648–52.

Kamar, G. & Argos, P. (1984). Primary structural comparisons of RNA-dependent polymerases from plants, animals and bacterial viruses. *Nucleic Acids Research* **12**, 7269–82.

Larder, B. A., Purifoy, D. J. M., Powell, K. L. & Darby, G., (1987a). Site-specific mutagenesis of AIDS virus reverse transcriptase. *Nature* **327**, 716–7.

Larder, B. A., Purifoy, D. J. M., Powell, K. & Darby, G. (1987b). AIDS virus reverse transcriptase defined by high level expression in *Escherichia coli*. *EMBO Journal* **6**, 3133–7.

Mitsuya, H. & Broder, S. (1987). Strategies for antiviral therapy in AIDS. *Nature* **325**, 773–8.

Tisdale, M., Ertl, P., Larder, B. A., Purifoy, D. J. M., Darby, G. & Powell, K. L. (1988). Characterization of HIV RT using monoclonal antibodies: The role of the C-terminus in antibody reactivity and enzyme function. *Journal of Virology,* in press.

Weiss, R., Teich, N., Varmus, H. & Coffin, J. Eds (1985). *RNA Tumour Viruses*, 2nd edn. Cold Spring Harbor Laboratories, Cold Spring Harbor, NY.

Journal of Antimicrobial Chemotherapy (1989) **23**, Suppl. A, 55–62

Strategies for the development of vaccines against HIV

Philip D. Minor

*National Institute for Biological Standards and Control,
Blanche Lane, South Mimms, Potters Bar, Herts EN6 3QG, UK*

Possible approaches to the development of vaccines against HIV are reviewed in the light of experience with existing virus vaccines and understanding of the process of viral infection. While HIV infection presents serious theoretical problems in developing vaccines most are also encountered in some form with other virus infections.

The very nature of HIV infection raises objections to using live attenuated or inactivated virus vaccines, as it is difficult to ensure that they are non-infectious or completely inactivated. The most promising types of vaccine involve expression of viral antigens in acceptable vectors either as virus vectors, or recombinant DNA products. However, the problem of identifying the antigen needed to induce adequate protective immunity remains and there is a clear need for a usable animal model to establish the potential of vaccines for human use.

Introduction

Vaccination has proved a highly successful strategy in the control of a range of diseases caused by viruses, including smallpox, yellow fever and poliomyelitis, and is one of the obvious routes in attempting to control AIDS. In recent years developments in recombinant DNA technology and understanding of immunological processes have suggested new routes to the production of vaccines, including those against diseases where the efficacy of existing vaccines is questionable. However, the prospects for the development of an effective vaccine may well depend on the pathogen concerned, its mode of spread and the rapidity with which it adapts to the host, as well as on the immune system of the host.

Human immunodeficiency virus (HIV) is transmitted in body fluids, and is a retrovirus capable of integration into the genome of the host cell, which may produce the symptoms of AIDS several years after the initial infection. Moreover, it infects the cells which mount the immune response, appears to be capable of rapid antigenic change especially in its surface proteins which may be considered the first target of a protective immune response, and is also believed to be capable of transmission directly from cell to cell without the release of free virus; this may indeed be the most effective mode of transmission. Many of these features of the virus appear to raise doubts about the possibility of effective vaccination; for example, the integration of the viral genome into the genome of the host cell suggests that the virus may become latent, and that a vaccine must thus be able to prevent even the first round of viral replication in an infected individual. This is a severe challenge, but possible parallels exist in other vaccines. For example, varicella virus is able to integrate into the host cell genome, but an effective vaccine is in use in the USA. The varicella vaccine is a live attenuated strain, which for many reasons may be an inappropriate path for an HIV vaccine. Thus it is not clear whether the vaccine strain itself integrates into the host genome and persists for life, something which would be highly undesirable for an HIV vaccine. However, it is valuable to review experience with existing vaccines as the theoretical objections to vaccination against HIV may have arisen and been dealt with to a greater or lesser extent in preparations against other viruses in current use. Moreover, the strategies used in the development of existing vaccines could form a model for the development of vaccines against HIV.

This paper considers some of the preparations in current use including live attenuated vaccines, whole killed vaccines and subunit vaccines consisting of a single viral polypeptide which may be obtained either from the virus directly or by recombinant DNA technology. Experimental vaccines including genetically engineered live virus vectors, chemically defined synthetic peptides and anti-idiotypes will be discussed, and the relevance of the existing and experimental vaccines to HIV considered. The types of vaccine considered possible currently are indicated in Table I.

Table I. Possible types of viral vaccine

Type	Current example	Applicability to HIV
Live attenuated virus	polio, mumps, measles, rubella, yellow fever, smallpox	no
Killed virus	polio, influenza	unlikely
Recombinant protein	hepatitis B	yes
Live virus vector (vaccinia, adenovirus etc.)	none in use, several known to protect animals	possible
Peptides	none—protection data limited	possible
Anti-idiotype	none—protection data very limited	possible

Inactivated vaccines against influenza

Influenza vaccines have been available and in use for forty years. Their impact on overall morbidity has been negligible, although they are of considerable value in specific target groups such as chronic bronchitics or asthmatics. In the western world non-infectious vaccines are used exclusively, including inactivated virus and protein subunit vaccines. Estimates of the effectiveness of the vaccines in protecting from disease vary from only 40% to 80% (Williams *et al.*, 1973) and it is not clearly established whether the lack of impact of vaccination is due to failure to use the vaccine on a sufficient scale, or to a defect in the strategy of vaccination as applied to influenza. Perhaps most importantly influenza undergoes two types of antigenic variation which may handicap the effectiveness of vaccination. Antigenic shift involves the alteration *en bloc* of the major antigen involved in the protective response, a process believed to occur as a result of genomic reassortment with another influenza virus. The process of antigenic shift leads to the generation of a totally novel strain to which the human population has little immunity. It therefore results in a global epidemic or pandemic of influenza. However, influenza is also able to undergo antigenic drift, a process generally believed to involve the accumulation of point mutations. This leads to the development of new epidemic strains (Wiley, Wilson & Skehel, 1981) responsible for more limited outbreaks. It can be shown that individuals infected by a pandemic strain can be infected subsequently by a second strain derived from it by a process of antigenic drift (Davies, Grilli & Smith, 1986) which correlates with observations of influenza epidemics caused by variants of a single pandemic strain, which occur at intervals of a few years. Vaccines are evaluated annually to ensure that the strains included are representative of the circulating strains. However, a long term study in the specialized environment of a boarding school in the UK suggested that this strategy may not be adequate (Hoskins *et al.*, 1979). The findings indicated that while the first vaccination afforded 80% protection against challenge, as found in other studies, revaccination of these individuals with subsequent updated strains provided negligible protection. The reasons for this are not clear.

Experience with influenza thus indicates that antigenic variability in viruses may cause considerable problems, which may not be surmountable even by successive vaccinations with antigenically different strains.

As HIV, the causative agent of AIDS, appears to undergo major variation in its major surface antigen, it is possible that similar difficulties may be encountered in developing an effective HIV vaccine.

Live attenuated vaccines against poliomyelitis

Oral polio vaccines are among the safest and most efficacious vaccines used in the developed world. The virus strains used have remained the same for nearly thirty years, confirming the general view that wild-type polioviruses do not undergo significant antigenic drift. This raises the possibility that the virus is basically invariant, which would be consistent with the high degree of safety associated with the live vaccines strains (Nkowane *et al.*, 1987) despite the fact that they may proliferate for prolonged periods in the intestinal tracts of recipients. In fact it has been shown that the virus may evolve rapidly. Thus viruses may undergo rapid change during epidemics (Nottay *et al.*, 1981). It has been shown that only two mutations account for the greater part of the attenuated phenotype of the Sabin type 3 strain of poliovirus vaccine (Westrop *et al.*, 1987) and that at least one of these reverts to the virulent genotype very rapidly as the virus proliferates in the human gut (Evans *et al.*, 1985). Other extensive genetic changes have been shown to occur regularly in healthy vaccinees (Minor *et al.*, 1986) including recombination between different serotypes, point mutations in antigenic sites and other mutations of unknown effect. Such changes may occur in all vaccine recipients, and can include the loss of both mutations associated with the attenuated phenotype, although it is possible that other attenuating mutations are acquired in the course of recombination events. The proven antigenic stability of the virus and the extremely safe character of the oral polio vaccines are therefore not easily explained.

The efficacy of a vaccine may thus depend not only on the immunogenicity of a preparation, but also on the way in which the virus behaves in its natural environment. Factors involved in the growth of poliovirus in its host clearly make it relatively easy to develop vaccines which will prevent disease, but it is not clear what those factors are.

Subunit recombinant DNA vaccines against hepatitis B

Several antigens are detectable in individuals infected with hepatitis B virus, including surface antigen (HbSAg) core antigen (Hbc) and e antigen (Hbe). It was found that the development of antibodies to HbSAg was a good indication that the virus would be cleared from infected individuals; this antigen was thus the most likely candidate for a subunit vaccine. The blood of chronically infected individuals has high levels of surface antigen most of which is found in the form of particles 22 nm in diameter in which the only viral component is the protein corresponding to HbSAg. The first commercial vaccine against hepatitis B was thus prepared by purifying 22 nm particles from the blood of infected individuals, using procedures which would inactivate the infectious virus. This vaccine proved both highly efficacious (Szmuness et al., 1980) and extremely safe. The cost of production and hypothetical future supply problems led to the development of recombinant products in which the gene coding for the surface antigen was expressed in yeast. Two such products are currently in use and others are being developed, including one where the gene is expressed in mammalian cells. The viral protein produced associates with cellular lipid and assembles into a particle similar to that obtained directly with the virus and may be purified as such. Vaccines based on this material have been shown to be safe, to induce antibody and to interrupt transmission of hepatitis B from mother to child, the only ethically acceptable trial now possible. While the principle of a recombinant DNA subunit vaccine is thought to be generally applicable, hepatitis B remains the only one in current commercial use, and may be a useful model for HIV. Thus vaccines against hepatitis B began to be developed in earnest after a careful study of the immune responses in patients who were recovering; similar studies of HIV infected individuals not showing symptoms of AIDS may be as revealing (Pederson et al., 1987). In addition, the mode of transmission and the groups at highest risk are the same for hepatitis B and HIV.

New approaches to viral vaccines

In recent years novel approaches to the development of vaccines have been suggested as a consequence of developments in recombinant DNA technology, chemical synthesis and immunology. While some appear promising, only hepatitis B vaccine has reached the stage of commercial application. It has proved possible to delete substantial portions of the genomes of large DNA viruses such as poxviruses or adenoviruses, and insert segments of foreign DNA, including viral antigens such as rabies glycoprotein or HIV envelope glycoprotein. Provided the virus is still able to multiply adequately an individual infected with such modified viruses will generate an immune response to the foreign gene expressed. Such live vectors must be of acceptably low pathogenicity and not transmissible to others.

Viruses may also be used as vectors for production in vitro. The insect baculoviruses produce very large amounts of a single protein (the polyhedrin protein) when they infect their natural host. The gene encoding this protein can be replaced with an alternative gene by genetic engineering, after which the foreign gene will be produced in large amounts when the modified virus infects its host. Such viruses clearly will not be used to infect vaccinees themselves, but to produce material for subsequent purification.

The possibility of using chemically defined peptides as immunogens has been raised in a number of areas, including hepatitis B (Dreesman *et al.*, 1982) and influenza (Green *et al.*, 1982) but the only system in which a convincing protective immune response has been demonstrated is a peptide whose sequence is derived from foot and mouth disease virus (Bittle *et al.*, 1982). Current work in which the presentation of the peptide has been modified is encouraging (Clarke *et al.*, 1987).

The anti-idiotype approach is based on the view that an antibody binding site forms a negative image of the antigen to which it binds specifically. If the antibody is used as an antigen in turn, the antibodies which will recognize it should resemble the initial antigen. Such second antibodies, known as anti-idiotypes could in principle be used in place of the antigen. This has been reported for rabies (Reagan *et al.*, 1987) and for hepatitis B (Kennedy *et al.*, 1984) but the approach remains speculative.

Several novel methods of presentation of antigens and novel adjuvants not yet used for commercial vaccine production are being pursued. Though these studies and others are of considerable general importance, one of the main difficulties of vaccine production remains, and that is the initial identification of the antigen needed to induce adequate protective immunity.

Relevance of HIV structure and epidemiology to vaccine development

Information on the clinical aspects of HIV infection and AIDS is limited to the past ten years. As several years may elapse between infection and the development of AIDS, clinical and epidemiological aspects of the disease relevant to vaccination remain unclear. The number of infected individuals who will ultimately develop immune deficiency, is not known although it is expected to be high. While it is generally assumed from experience to date, and by analogy with related virus infections in animals that infected individuals will be unable to clear the virus, this is not established. These and other factors make the assessment of hypothetical vaccines potentially difficult.

The virus resembles lentiviruses such as visna-maedi virus of sheep, caprine arthritis virus and infectious equine anaemia. It possesses reverse transcriptase activity and the ability to integrate into the host genome where it may remain unexpressed and therefore inaccessible to the immune system. The extent to which integration is a necessary function for virus growth is unknown.

It is established that one of the most effective ways of infecting individuals is by transfusion of whole cells, and *in vitro* it appears that effective transmission may be from cell to cell. This would involve the fusion of infected and uninfected cells so that infection would not necessarily require free virus. This is often cited as a major obstacle to the development of effective vaccines against HIV. There is a parallel in conventional vaccines, however, in that measles may also be transmitted directly from cell to cell, yet existing live vaccines are highly effective at preventing disease. In contrast the early measles vaccines were based on inactivated virus, and the process of preparation destroyed the immunogenicity of the fusion protein responsible for cell to cell spread. Vaccine recipients were thus protected in so far as infection involved free virus, but were not protected from cellular transmission, and developed severe symptoms as a result. This experience underlines the need to understand the virological basis of disease if non-infectious vaccines are to be used, but also indicates that cellular transmission can be prevented effectively.

A further potentially serious obstacle is that while an infected individual mounts an immune response to a large number of the viral proteins, there is as yet no indication that the development of antibodies to any particular protein results in clearance of the viral infection. The example of hepatitis B may be of value, where high levels of antibody specific for the core proteins may occur unassociated with recovery from disease, but antibody specific for the surface antigen is a good indication of recovery, as outlined previously. In the context of HIV, studies on the declining levels of antibodies directed to the core protein (gag) corresponding with a rise in antigenaemia as individuals progress from being infected to developing disease may be of significance (Pedersen et al., 1987). If anti-gag antibody levels were maintained, disease might be averted although the individual might remain infected (Salk, 1987).

Genetic antigenic variation in HIV has been described in some detail (Hahn et al., 1986). Much of this variation occurs in the envelope glycoprotein (env) and the genomic sequence of isolates made from an individual over a period of time, or from an individual at the same time may vary considerably. This would suggest that, as in the case of influenza, antigenic variation may present difficulties if a protective immune response must be directed to the envelope glycoprotein.

The long period between infection and the development of immune deficiency makes it difficult to establish the clinical and epidemiological factors which are of particular relevance to vaccine development. The existence of a relevant animal model would greatly assist these studies; it could be established for instance, whether immunity to infection or disease can ever be induced and maintained. Possible animal models include chimpanzees, which may be infected with HIV, and monkeys which may be infected by SIV, a related but distinct virus, which appears to produce similar symptoms in appropriate monkeys to those induced by HIV in man.

The possible types of vaccine which could be envisaged include attenuated live virus preparations. This could be based on an existing strain which produced infection without causing disease, or could be produced by a defined genetic engineering approach. Thus if the integrase function is not needed for virus replication, it might be deleted producing a virus capable of acute but not chronic infection. The strongest objection to such vaccines is that they cannot be tested. It is unlikely that a strain of HIV could be identified which could be confidently shown to be fully and permanently attenuated for man by in vitro tests, or tests in animals and thus be suitable as a candidate vaccine. The experience with oral polio vaccines outlined previously illustrates the potential problems in extrapolating from the retention or loss of attenuating markers to the suitability of a vaccine for use. The prolonged period between infection with HIV and the development of immune deficiency would in practice make it difficult to establish that the candidate vaccine strain was attenuated at all. It is therefore unlikely that any live vaccine based on an attenuated strain of HIV could ever be used.

Vaccines based on whole inactivated virus are potentially more acceptable. In practice it may be difficult to ensure that the virus is inactivated; the Cutter incident in the 1950s involving poorly inactivated polio vaccines caused many cases of poliomyelitis, and outbreaks of foot and mouth disease are occasionally traced to incompletely inactivated vaccines. The infectivity of these viruses, in contrast to that of HIV, is readily assayed. A final consideration involves the definition of inactivation; it is possible that the virus may be rendered non-infectious by most criteria in cell culture, but remain able to integrate into the host cell genome *in vivo*, thus initially establishing a latent infection.

The use of inactivated preparations in model systems, in contrast to their use in man, is likely to provide essential information in the development of vaccines, not least in establishing whether infection or immunodeficiency can be prevented by immunization. However, in practice the most promising type of vaccine for human use currently appears to involve the expression of viral antigens in acceptable vectors. Most work has so far focused on the envelope glycoprotein, because the equivalent protein in many other systems, including other retroviruses, is the target of neutralizing antibody. Results in chimpanzees have not been encouraging. Animals immunized with envelope glycoprotein (gp120) prepared from infected cells or appropriate vectors develop antibodies which do not satisfactorily neutralize the virus *in vitro* and do not protect the animals from infection with challenge virus. It can be argued, however, that the chimpanzee is an imperfect model for human AIDS as individual animals, though infected, have not been shown to develop AIDS-like symptoms. The *env* gene has been inserted into vaccinia and other live virus vectors and in one case the construct has been administered to humans resulting in antibody production. The protective efficacy, if any, of such a preparation remains to be seen. The other likely viral protein is the *gag* gene and there is much interest in it currently.

Other work in progress includes the identification of immunogenic peptides. Anti-idiotype technology has involved generating antibodies specific for the cellular receptor for the virus, and then generating anti-idiotypes to this. Neutralizing antibodies have been generated in this way and the hope is that they will involve a portion of the virus required for its virological function and thus be totally conserved between strains.

Conclusion

Vaccine development involves a combination of knowledge and effort from the disciplines of virology and immunology. Historically it has not been necessary to understand the mechanism by which vaccines work in order to develop them, but there appear to be relevant lessons to be learned from previous experience in the task of devising vaccines against HIV. In particular the nature of the virus imposes constraints on the kinds of vaccine which may be thought acceptable and there is a clear need for a usable animal model to establish the potential of vaccines for human use.

References

Bittle, J. L., Houghten, R. A., Alexander, H., Shinnick, T. M., Sutcliffe, J. G., Lerner, R. A. *et al.* (1982). Protection against foot and mouth disease by immunisation with a chemically synthesised peptide predicted from the viral nucleotide sequence. *Nature* **298**, 30–3.

Clarke, B. E., Newton, S. E., Carroll, A. R., Francis, M. J., Appleyard, G., Syred, A. D. *et al.* (1987). Improved immunogenicity of a peptide epitope after fusion to hepatitis B core protein. *Nature* **330**, 381–4.

Davies, J. R., Grilli, E. A. & Smith, A. J. (1986). Infection with influenza A H1N1. The effect of past experience on natural challenge. *Journal of Hygiene* **96**, 345–52.

Dreesman, G. R., Sanchez, Y., Ionescu-Matiu, I., Sparrow, J. T., Six, H. R., Peterson, D. L. *et al.*, (1982). Antibody to hepatitis B surface antigen after a single inoculation of uncoupled synthetic HBsAg peptides. *Nature* **295**, 158–60.

Evans, D. M. A., Dunn, G., Minor, P. D., Schild, G. C., Cann, A. J., Stanway, G. *et al.* (1985). A single nucleotide change in the 5′ non-coding region of the genome of the Sabin type 3 poliovaccine is associated with increased neurovirulence. *Nature* **314**, 548–50.

Green, N., Alexander, H., Olson, A., Alexander, S., Shinnick, T. M., Sutcliffe, J. G. *et al.* (1982). Immunogenic structure of the influenza virus haemagglutinin. *Cell* **28**, 477–87.

Hahn, B. H., Shaw, G. M., Taylor, M. E., Redfield, R. R., Markham, P. D., Salahuddin, S. Z., *et al.* (1986). Genetic variation in HTLV3/LAV over time in patients with AIDS or at risk for AIDS. *Science* **232**, 1548–53.

Hoskins, T. W., Davies, J. R., Smith, A. J., Miller, C. L. & Allchin, A. (1979). Assessment of inactivated influenza A vaccine after three outbreaks of influenza A at Christ's Hospital. *Lancet i*, 33–5.

Kennedy, R. C., Sparrow, J. T., Sanchez, Y., Melnick, J. L. & Dreesman, G. R., (1984). Enhancement of the immune response to a cyclic synthetic HBsAg peptide by prior injection of anti-idiotype antibodies. In *Modern Approaches to Vaccines: Molecular and Chemical Basis of Virus Virulence and Immunogenicity* (Channock, R. M. & Lerner, R. A., Eds), pp. 427–30. Cold Spring Harbor.

Minor, P. D., John, A., Ferguson, M. & Icenogle, J. P. (1986). Antigenic and molecular evolution of the vaccine strain of type 3 poliovirus during the period of excretion by a primary vaccinee. *Journal of General Virology* **67**, 693–706.

Nkowane, B. M., Wassilak, S. G. F., Orenstein, W. A., Bart, K., Schonberger, L. B., Hinman, A. R. *et al.* (1987). Vaccine-associated paralytic poliomyelitis. United States: 1973 through 1984. *Journal of the American Medical Association* **257**, 1335–40.

Nottay, B. K., Kew, O. M., Hatch, M. H., Heyward, J. T. & Obijeski, J. F. (1981). Molecular variation of type 1 vaccine related and wild polioviruses during replication in humans. *Virology* **108**, 405–23.

Pedersen, C., Moller-Nielson, C., Vestergaard, B. F., Gerstoft, J., Krogsgaard, K. & Nielsen, J. O. (1987). Temporal relation of antigenaemia and loss of antibodies to core antigens to development of clinical disease in HIV infection. *British Medical Journal* **295**, 567–9.

Reagan, K. J., Wunner, W. H., Wiktor, T. J. & Koprowski, H. (1983). Anti-idiotypic antibodies induce neutralising antibodies to rabies virus glycoprotein. *Journal of Virology* **48**, 660–6.

Salk, J. (1987). Prospects for the control of AIDS by immunising seropositive individuals. *Nature* **327**, 473–6.

Szmuness, W., Stevens, C. E., Harley, E. J., Zang, E. A., Oleszko, W. R., Williams, D. C. *et al.* (1980). Hepatitis B vaccine; demonstration of efficacy in controlled clinical trial in a high risk population in the United States. *New England Journal of Medicine* **303**, 833–41.

Westrop, G. D., Evans, D. M. A., Minor, P. D., Magrath, D. I., Schild, G. C. & Almond, J. W. (1987). Investigation of the molecular basis of attenuation in the Sabin type 3 vaccine using novel recombinant polioviruses constructed from infections cDNA. In *The Molecular Biology of the Positive Strand RNA Viruses, FEMS Symposium,* No. 32 (Rowlands, D. J., Mayo, M. A. & Mahy, B. W. J., Eds), pp. 53–60. Academic Press, London.

Wiley, D. C., Wilson, I. A. & Skehel, J. J. (1981). Structural identification of the antibody binding sites of Hong Kong influenza haemagglutinin and their involvement in antigenic variation. *Nature* **289**, 373–8.

Williams, M. C., Davignon, L., McDonald, J. C., Pavilaris, P. V., Bondreault, A. & Clayton, A. J. (1973). Trials of aqueous killed influenza vaccine in Canada, 1968–69. *Bulletin of the World Health Organisation* **49**, 333–40.

Journal of Antimicrobial Chemotherapy (1989) **23**, 63–65

Antimicrobial therapy of infections in patients with AIDS—an overview

Merle A. Sande

Medical Service, San Francisco General Hospital, 1001 Potrero Avenue, San Francisco, California 94110, USA

Introduction

The acquired immunodeficiency syndrome (AIDS) has clearly illustrated the critical role played by an intact cellular immune system in the successful chemotherapy of many infections. Infectious diseases physicians have become secure in their approach to antimicrobial therapy since administration of selective drugs, available for most infections, while static, are not in and of themselves 'cidal'. These bacteriostatic agents often forget that most drugs used to treat fungal, protozoan, and, more recently, viral infections, while static, are not in and of themselves 'cidal. These bacteriostatic agents usually require an intact, or relatively effective, cellular immune (monocyte-macrophage) system to ensure that the infecting organism(s) is eradicated and relapse prevented—an immune system which, in patients with AIDS, is neither intact nor relatively effective.

The need for maintenance therapy

Gradually we are learning that successful management of the various opportunistic infections that complicate the course of patients with AIDS requires an approach similar to that employed by oncologists in treating patients with malignancies. Initially, an induction phase, using full conventional-dose antimicrobial therapy, is used to control the acute infection, ameliorate symptoms, and reduce organism titres. However, if conventional drugs are used for only the duration that typically ensures cure in non-AIDS patients, relapse will often occur after therapy is discontinued. Thus, it is usually necessary to follow the induction phase of treatment with chronic suppressive or maintenance chemotherapy. This may be accomplished by using either the same drug that was used in the induction phase but in a lower dose or with less frequent administration, or another less toxic drug, or one that can be administered orally.

Pneumocystis pneumonia

This approach is now widely employed in treating patients with *Pneumocystis carinii* pneumonia (PCP), an illness that occurs in more than 80% of AIDS patients. Historically, PCP, when a complication of corticosteroid therapy or in patients with haematological malignancies (patients in whom there exists a less severe impairment of the cellular immune response than exists in patients with AIDS), could be cured with a two- to three-week course of pentamidine or high-dose parenteral trimethoprim-sulphamethoxazole. If this approach is taken with AIDS patients, up to 50 per cent of them will relapse in the six- to nine-month period following discontinuation of therapy (Kovacs & Masur, 1988). If maintenance therapy is employed, however, relapse rates can be reduced to less than 5 per cent (Fischl et al., 1988). Most maintenance regimens that have been tested appear to be effective, including therapy with orally administered trimethoprim-sulphamethoxazole, pyrimethamine-sulfadoxine (Fansidar), or inhaled aerosolized pentamidine.

Toxoplasmosis

A similar response has been documented in AIDS patients with central nervous system toxoplasmosis, another protozoan infection, and one which is activated in the AIDS patient when his T_4 cell count drops and severe impairment in cellular immunity occurs. Patients with this infection, which typically presents as a mass lesion(s) in the brain, respond remarkably well to oral therapy with sulphadiazine and pyrimethamine. The mass lesion will usually improve or disappear completely (as judged by computed tomographic scanning) with therapy, but, if therapy is discontinued, reappearance of the lesion or relapse will occur in most patients. Therefore, maintenance therapy is recommended (Luft & Remington, 1988).

Fungal infections

Patients with opportunistic fungal infections also follow a similar pattern. Cryptococcal meningitis is an extremely common infection in the AIDS patient; more than 150 cases of this infection have been treated at San Francisco General Hospital since 1981 (Chuck, S. L., personal communication). Amphotericin B, 0·5–0·8 mg/kg/day iv, is highly effective in ameliorating symptoms, producing a drop in cryptococcal antigen titres, and eliminating cryptococci from the cerebrospinal fluid. However, if a six- to ten-week course of therapy (which is adequate to cure the vast majority of cryptococcal infections in non-AIDS patients) is administered to AIDS patients, relapse will occur in most of them (Dismukes, 1988). Various maintenance regimens, including amphotericin, 1 mg/kg iv once a week (a regimen that appears to be quite effective, although published data are sparse), have been employed. Based on our experience, we have found orally administered ketoconazole to be less effective. It is hoped that fluconazole, a new imidazole derivative with excellent activity against cryptococci and excellent penetration into the cerebrospinal fluid, will prove useful in this setting.

Another fungal infection that may be reactivated when the cellular immune system is destroyed by the human immunodeficiency virus (HIV) is caused by Histoplasma capsulatum. Reactivation of histoplasmal infection leads to widespread dissemination of the organism to the lungs, liver, spleen, lymph nodes, and bone marrow. Systemic response to conventional (induction phase) doses of amphotericin is good, but relapse is common after therapy is discontinued (Graybill, 1988). Ketoconazole appears to constitute effective maintenance therapy for preventing relapses. We have observed patients who, because they "felt so good," discontinued maintenance therapy after a year and subsequently relapsed within three weeks.

Bacterial infections

Interestingly, certain bacterial infections follow the same pattern of response to antimicrobial therapy. AIDS patients seem to be particularly susceptible to bacteraemia caused by non-typhoidal strains of the genus *Salmonella* (Celum *et al.*, 1987). Although the salmonella bacteraemia is cleared rapidly with therapy with ampicillin, trimethoprim-sulphamethoxazole, chloramphenicol, or ceftriaxone, bacteraemia with associated fever and chills usually recurs when therapy is discontinued. We have successfully used orally administered ciprofloxacin, 750 mg bid, as maintenance or suppressive therapy to control salmonella infections in patients with AIDS (Hahn, S. M., Gerberding, J. L. & Sande, M. A., unpublished work). In two cases in which ciprofloxacin was discontinued after several months, relapse occurred within three weeks.

Viral infections

A similar approach has been necessary to control retinitis caused by cytomegalovirus, a progressive infection that may lead to blindness in patients with AIDS. Ganciclovir (DHPG) administered intravenously usually stops progression of retinal destruction and in some cases leads to regression of concomitant oedema and visual impairment (Drew, 1988). If therapy with ganciclovir is discontinued after a two-week induction period, the progressive retinitis resumes, but can usually be controlled with maintenance therapy consisting of periodic ganciclovir administration (Drew, 1988).

Conclusion

From experience with these diverse infections, a repeating pattern is emerging. Most of the opportunistic infections that complicate AIDS are incurable, at least with currently available antimicrobial therapy. Nonetheless, by aggressively treating the acute disease, the infection can be controlled and the suffering of the patient reduced. Relapse can be minimized by managing the patient with maintenance or suppressive therapy. It appears that we might have learned a valuable lesson here from our oncologist colleagues.

References

Celum, C. L., Chaisson, R. E., Rutherford, G. W., Barnhart, J. L. & Echenberg, D. F. (1987). Incidence of salmonellosis in patients with AIDS. *Journal of Infectious Diseases* **156,** 998–1002.

Dismukes, W. E. (1988). Cryptococcal meningitis in patients with AIDS. *Journal of Infectious Diseases* **157,** 624–8.

Drew, W. L. (1988). What is the clinical impact of CMV infection in patients with AIDS? *Journal of Infectious Diseases* **158,** 449–56.

Fischl, M. A., Dickinson, G. M. & La Voie, L. (1988). Safety and efficacy of sulfamethoxazole and trimethoprim chemoprophylaxis for *Pneumocystis carinii* pneumonia in AIDS. *Journal of the American Medical Association* **259,** 1185–9.

Graybill, J. R. (1988). Histoplasmosis in the setting of AIDS. *Journal of Infectious Diseases* **158,** 623–6.

Kovacs, J. A. & Masur, H. (1988). *Pneumocystis carinii* pneumonia: therapy and prophylaxis. *Journal of Infectious Diseases* **158,** 254–9.

Luft, B. J. & Remington, J. S. (1988). Toxoplasmic encephalitis. *Journal of Infectious Diseases* **157,** 1–6.

Journal of Antimicrobial Chemotherapy (1989) **23**, *Suppl. A*, 67–75

Pneumocystis carinii pneumonia and its treatment in patients with AIDS

B. G. Gazzard

St Stephen's Hospital, Fulham Road, Chelsea, London, SW10 9TH, UK

Pneumocystis carinii pneumonia (PCP) is the commonest opportunistic infection in AIDS patients. The diagnosis should be strongly suspected in patients who are cyanosed and who present with interstitial pneumonia.

The management of PCP in AIDS patients is very similar to that in other groups with the same infection. Trimethoprim-sulphamethoxazole (TMP/SMZ) combinations or pentamidine remain the therapies of choice. Side effects of TMP/SMZ are much greater in AIDS patients than in other immuno-suppressed patients and are similar in frequency to those of pentamidine. Occasionally, pentamidine produces life-threatening complications. Trimetrexate with folinic acid is likely to be as effective against pneumocystis as the two first-line drugs and trimethoprim/dapsone combinations can be given orally and are clearly effective in moderately severe infections. Prophylaxis following an attack of PCP undoubtedly reduces the risk of re-infection, but may not materially alter the overall prognosis. The best drug regimen remains controversial but fortnightly inhaled pentamidine has the advantage of patient acceptability and very low risk of side-effects.

Introduction

Pneumocystis carinii pneumonia (PCP) was initially described in debilitated premature babies (Ivady & Paldy, 1958). As antibodies to *Pneumocystis carinii* appear in the first few years of life it appears that most humans are exposed to this infection over this period. PCP occurs in congenital immune deficiency states and in adults following immunosuppressive therapy (Western, Perera & Shultz, 1970). The epidemic of AIDS was first recognised as a result of PCP appearing in a group of homosexuals with no apparent reason for an immune deficit (Gottlieb *et al.*, 1981). Pneumocystis remains the commonest opportunist encountered in AIDS patients, establishing the diagnosis of AIDS in 55% of cases and occurring at some time during the illness in 80% (Wofsy, 1987). Rational therapy for PCP has been hampered by the inability to grow the organism *in vitro* and doubts about the relevance of rodent models to human experience.

Clinical presentation

Dry cough, fever and shortness of breath are the classic clinical presentations, although the disease is more insidious in those patients with AIDS, with a median time to diagnosis from onset of symptoms of 25 days compared with 5 days in patients who develop PCP as a result of immunosuppressive therapy (Kovacs *et al.*, 1984). The most important symptom which should alert the clinician is shortness of breath, which

0305–7453/89/23A067 + 09 $02.00/0

is rare in most other respiratory ailments affecting this age group. The sparsity of physical signs in the chest is in contrast to the sometimes severe cyanosis. The partial pressure of oxygen may be normal in about 10% of cases but is usually reduced and in our series the mortality was directly related to the mean arterial partial pressure of oxygen on arrival in hospital, with a 50% mortality for those with a partial pressure of oxygen of less than 6 KPa (Gazzard, Anderson & Gardner, 1987) (Figure 1).

Diagnosis

The combination of interstitial lung infiltration and hypoxia in a patient who is HIV positive is so strongly suggestive of the diagnosis that some authors have suggested that treatment should be started empirically and further investigations be limited to those who fail to respond (Pozniak et al., 1986). Certainly the rapidly growing number of cases and the eventual poor prognosis indicate a need to define less invasive techniques for confirming the diagnosis. In 1981 and 1982 many patients in the United States underwent open lung biopsy, but now the standard investigations are bronchoscopy, with broncho-alveolar lavage (BAL), with or without transbronchial biopsy (TBB). A comparison of the sensitivity of BAL and TBB is hampered by there being no definitive diagnostic test for PCP and variable laboratory expertise in different centres. Staining of sputum, induced by breathing hypertonic saline (3%), for

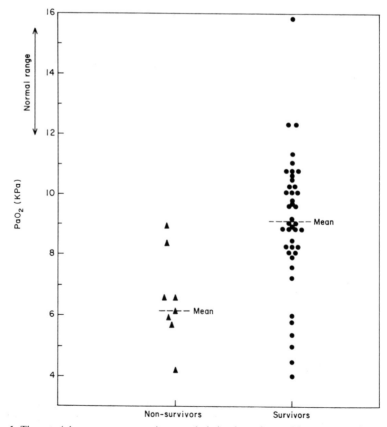

Figure 1. The arterial oxygen concentration on admission in patients with pneumocystis pneumonia.

cysts of pneumocystis might reduce the need for bronchoscopy, but although good results have been obtained in some units, we have found it difficult to produce sputum samples in the majority of our patients (Editorial, 1986).

Patients with no hypoxia and/or a normal chest X-ray who are febrile and short of breath are the most difficult group to diagnose. Although they often respond to a course of treatment for PCP, such patients are less likely to have PCP diagnosed successfully by TBB. It is not clear whether such patients do not have PCP or have too few protozoa in the lungs to be detected in small biopsy samples. Gallium scanning appears to be a sensitive but non-specific test in these patients, but is not readily available in many hospitals. We have used an ear oximeter to measure oxygen desaturation in response to exercise in patients with a normal resting blood oxygen tension. Desaturation occurred in all but one of the patients who subsequently had proven PCP on bronchoscopy (Figure 2).

Treatment

Specific dilemmas in AIDS patients

It was fortunate that at the start of the AIDS epidemic successful treatment for PCP had already been developed. While the search for successful antiviral agents is

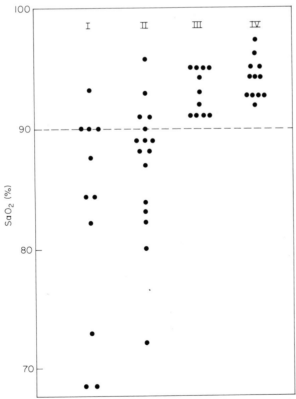

Figure 2. The oxygen desaturation produced by exercise measured using an ear oximeter in patients who had pneumocystic pneumonia with (I) or without (II) arterial hypoxia at rest, a group of patients with lung infections other than PCP (III) and a group of controls (IV).

understandably arousing most research interest, in the short term the prognosis of AIDS is likely to be improved by successful management of opportunistic infections. In AIDS the annual attack rate for PCP is greater than 30%, in contrast to renal transplants, leukaemia and lymphoma, where it appears to be between 0·01 and 1% (Kovaks *et al.,* 1984). Short term survival following PCP is now 74% in the largest series of treated AIDS patients, but this is reduced to between 40% and 60% in subsequent episodes of infection (Tuazon & Labriola, 1987).

Unresolved questions in PCP treatment include the most efficacious initial therapy, the duration of such treatment, the route of administration, the effectiveness of prophylaxis against the initial attack and to prevent relapse, and the role if any of mechanical ventilation.

Experience with treatment of PCP in non-AIDS patients

Pentamidine isethionate has been used for more than 30 years in the treatment of African trypanosomiasis and was first used as a therapy against PCP in children in 1958 (Ivady & Paldy, 1958). By 1970, experience with 164 patients had been reported with a survival rate of about 50% and side effects in about 40% of patients (Western *et al.,* 1970). Initially pentamidine was administered by intramuscular injection, but sterile abscesses were a frequent complication and the drug is now usually given by slow intravenous infusion over an hour. More rapid injection may result in profound hypotension.

In 1974, success in treating a rodent model of PCP with a trimethoprim-sulphamethoxazole combination (TMP/SMZ) was reported and by 1980 sufficient clinical experience had accumulated to conclude that this was the preferred method of treatment (Winston *et al.,* 1980). An overall response rate of 67% in 88 patients was reported, which rose to 85·5% in those treated for more than nine days. TMP/SMZ was recommended as initial treatment for PCP because side effects only occurred in 13% of patients, indicating a better toxic therapeutic ratio than for pentamidine.

In 1984 Kovacs and his colleagues carried out a comparison of therapy in AIDS (49 patients) and non-AIDS patients (39 patients) with PCP (Kovacs *et al.,* 1984). The AIDS patients had a significantly longer duration of illness, a lower respiratory rate and a higher mean arterial oxygen tension. The overall survival rate in the two groups was identical, but while adverse reactions to pentamidine were equally frequent in both groups, and similar to previous experience, side effects with TMP/SMZ were much more common in AIDS patients. This observation has been confirmed repeatedly and about 60% of AIDS patients will react adversely to this combination Wharton *et al.,* 1986). Skin rashes in 29% of AIDS patients and neutropenia in 46% are particularly common, although rarely described in non-AIDS patients. It has been suggested that all patients given TMP/SMZ should also be treated with folinic acid (Kinzie & Taylor, 1984). Pneumocystis organisms lack transport systems for reduced folic acid and thus folinic acid has no effect on the efficacy of TMP/SMZ. However, there is no evidence that bone marrow suppression is related to folic acid deficiency.

Initial therapy for PCP in AIDS patients (Table I)

Trimethoprim-sulphamethoxazole and pentamidine

As there is no advantage in the use of TMP/SMZ in terms of toxic side effects in AIDS patients, the problems of which agent to use first remains unresolved. In a prospective

Table I. Treatment of pneumocystis carinii pneumonia

Drug	Dose and route	Duration	Side effects
Co-trimoxazole (TMP-SMZ)	40 ml of intravenous solution (480 mg in 5 ml) diluted in 1 litre of normal saline twice daily. Or eight adult tablets (480 mg each) twice daily	14–21 days	Fever, rash, nausea, vomiting, marrow suppression, abnormal liver function tests
Pentamidine	4 mg pentamidine isethionate or 2·3 mg/kg pentamidine base per day given intravenously diluted in 250 ml of 5% dextrose	14 days	Hypotension, rash, nausea, vomiting, nephrotoxicity, hypoglycaemia, thrombocytopenia
	or		
	600 mg pentamidine isethionate in 6 ml sterile water inhaled via a nebuliser daily	14 days	Bronchospasm
Eflornithine	400 mg/kg/day by continuous intravenous infusion followed	14 days	Diarrhoea, thrombocytopenia, leucopenia
Dapsone and trimethoprim	100 mg/day as a single oral dose. 20 mg/kg/day intravenously or orally in four divided doses	21 days	Nausea, vomiting, haemolytic anaemia, methaemoglobinaemia, rash, leucopenia, abnormal liver function tests
Trimetrexate	30 mg/m²/day as an intravenous bolus	21 days	Leucopenia, thrombocytopenia, abnormal liver function tests
plus folinic acid	20 mg/m²/6-hourly as an intravenous bolus or orally	23 days	Rash, nephrotoxicity
with or without sulphadiazine	1 g every 6 h orally	21 days	Rash, leucopenia

randomized trial, 21 patients received TMP/SMZ as initial therapy and 20 pentamidine. Five of the former group died and one of the latter, although the mortality by three months was identical (Wharton *et al.*, 1986). Although this was a small study subject to a high type-II error, subsequent workers re-analyzing the data have suggested a clear trend in favour of pentamidine as initial therapy (Erban, 1987). This is in contrast to the findings in non-AIDS patients (Winston *et al.*, 1980). In Wharton's study, 10 of the 20 patients treated with TMP/SMZ and 11 of the 20 patients treated with pentamidine had a major drug reaction requiring a change of therapy (Wharton *et al.*, 1986). Although the frequency of drug reactions to both drugs in AIDS patients is similar, the consequences of side effects with pentamidine may be more serious. Leucopenia is the commonest reaction to pentamidine followed by a rise in blood urea. Both of these are reversible on cessation of therapy. More importantly, hypoglycaemia and pancreatitis, although unusual, may be life-threatening complications of pentamidine therapy.

Oral dapsone and trimethoprim

Other regimens have also been used for the treatment of PCP. Dapsone is a sulphone which competes with para-amino benzoic acid in folic acid synthesis. A combination of oral dapsone and trimethoprim was as effective as TMP/SMZ in a rat model of pneumocystis and so was used in an open study in humans (Leoung *et al.*, 1986). This study, which excluded those patients 'likely to die within one week without therapy' (12 patients), showed that 15 treated patients all improved, and only two had serious side effects necessitating stopping therapy. Minor side effects however were common, and patients with glucose 6 phosphate dehydrogenase deficiency were excluded. Although this open study, which excluded a number of patients, is unreliable in predicting the outcome of all patients treated with this regimen, massive increases in numbers of patients with PCP over the next few years indicate the urgent need for an effective oral therapy. The same group therefore compared oral TMP/SMZ with dapsone/trimethoprim in a randomized double blind study of 58 patients with moderate hypoxia (Medina *et al.*, 1987). Treatments failures occurred in only four patients (two from each group) but toxicity occurred in nearly half (24 patients), more commonly with the TMP/SMZ combination. Only a third of the patients needed to be in hospital because of symptoms, and the others could have been successfully managed from the outset at home, although all needed careful monitoring for toxicity in the second week of therapy.

Trimetrexate

Trimetrexate is a potent anti-folic acid drug developed as an anti-cancer agent which was shown to be 1500 times more potent an inhibitor of dihydrofolate reductase in *P. carinii* than trimethoprim (Allegra *et al.*, 1987). An open study of this drug in PCP was carried out using reduced folate (folinic acid) as a means of protecting the host tissues from the antifolate effects (Allegra *et al.*, 1987). Three groups of patients were studied, those failing to respond to standard therapy (16), those who had a history of sensitivity to sulphonamides (16), and a group treated with trimetrexate and sulphadiazine as initial therapy (17). Over 60% of all these groups improved with treatment and this response rate increased to 71% in those patients also treated with sulphadiazine. While this was not a controlled clinical trial, all patients, however sick, were included and a high proportion were treated for the second or third episode of PCP where the prognosis should be worse. Thus it is likely that trimetrexate represents an important additional agent in the treatment of PCP and may become the agent of first choice as the toxic effects were minimal and did not lead to cessation of therapy in any patient. It has recently been licensed by the Federal Drugs Administration for use in the United States.

Inhaled pentamidine

Pneumocystis organisms appear to be confined to the alveolar space in PCP. Inhaled pentamidine delivered via a nebuliser produces high alveolar concentrations of the drug in both man and mice, with negligible blood concentrations. The pentamidine levels in broncho-alveolar lavage specimens remain unaltered for at least 24 h after therapy (Montgomery *et al.*, 1987). This approach is likely to considerably reduce the toxic side effects of parental pentamidine, and has been used in open studies of 50 moderately ill patients with PCP (patients with an arterial PaO_2 of less than 50 mm of mercury at presentation were excluded). All but two of the patients responded and the only side effect was coughing. We have used this regimen in more seriously ill patients with PCP but in these it appears less effective. Data are required on the most efficient delivery system and on a comparison of inhaled pentamidine with other agents as initial therapy in moderately ill patients with PCP.

Eflornithine

Eflornithine is an inhibitor of ornithine decarboxylase, which is important in the synthesis of polyamines, necessary for cell growth. It shows activity against *P. carinii* and other protozoans. Its use in AIDS patients has so far been limited to salvage studies of patients who have failed to respond to initial therapy. In the largest series of 345 patients, 266 survived if they had received more than four days' therapy. Significantly, 23% of mechanically ventilated patients who were treated for more than 14 days, survived (McLees *et al.*, 1987). Such studies are difficult to evaluate in patients whose survival may be poor after failure of initial therapy, but our experience confirms that 60% of such patients do respond to eflornithine treatment. This drug needs further investigation as initial therapy for PCP. The spectrum of toxic effects includes frequent blood dyscrasias (most usually thrombocytopenia, in 48% of patients) and diarrhoea in 20% (particularly with oral therapy).

Corticosteroids

About 10% of patients with PCP have changes on X-ray suggestive of adult respiratory distress syndrome (Gazzard, B. G., Youle, M., Gardner, T. K., Gleeson, J. A., unpublished observations) and it has been suggested that the prognosis of seriously ill patients with PCP (PaO_2 less than 60 mm of mercury on admission) may be improved with the addition of methylprednisolone 40 mg 6-hourly for seven days (McFadden *et al.*, 1987). This study was uncontrolled but a striking improvement in survival (nine out of ten) was seen compared with two of eight survivors in the conventionally treated group. Similar results have been reported from France in an equally sick group of patients (Mottin *et al.*, 1987).

Prophylaxis

As the annual attack rate for PCP in AIDS patients is of the order of 30%, prophylaxis should be considered. Although pentamidine and TMP/SMZ are effective in treating PCP, the organism is frequently not eradicated and can be recovered at follow-up bronchoscopy. Whether or not the organisms are viable is unclear (Rosen *et al.*, 1983). Chemoprophylaxis against PCP should also be considered in high risk HIV antibody positive patients and those with Kaposi's sarcoma. High risk patients include those with a low OKT4 count, P24 antigen positivity in the blood, and loss of P24 antibody.

Early studies have shown that low dose oral daily TMP/SMZ is effective chemoprophylaxis against the development of PCP in high risk cancer patients (Hughes *et al.*, 1977). However, in one study of 28 patients with Kaposi's sarcoma randomised to receive placebo or TMP/SMZ, 12 of the 14 patients on active treatment were withdrawn because of side effects. The side effects of TMP/SMZ may be more acceptable in patients who have already suffered from an episode of PCP, partly because those who have shown hypersensitivity to TMP/SMZ will have been excluded. One published study demonstrated its effectiveness in long term survivors of PCP (greater than six months). None of 13 of a TMP/SMZ treated group developed PCP compared with 15 of the 19 placebo treated patients (Hollander, 1986). Prophylaxis, however, remains controversial as many of the treated patients died in a short period of other AIDS complications and the majority of the placebo group recovered following a full course of therapy.

An alternative prophylactic regimen of pyrimethamine/sulfadoxine (Fansidar) one tablet per week may also be effective and may be used cautiously, even in patients with TMP/SMZ hypersensitivity (Gottleib *et al.*, 1984). However, non-fatal episodes of Stevens-Johnson syndrome have been reported with this treatment (Navin *et al.*, 1985).

An alternative prophylactic regimen gaining widespread popularity is the use of inhaled pentamidine, either once weekly or fortnightly. The optimum dose, frequency of administration and effectiveness of such an approach have not been fully elucidated.

Influence of zidovudine

The original study of zidovudine chose survivors from PCP pneumonia as one of the entry criteria. Following zidovudine patients had fewer subsequent episodes of opportunistic infections including PCP, compared with those receiving placebo, and their survival was prolonged (Fischl *et al.*, 1987). In our experience in treating 155 patients with this drug, PCP is reduced in frequency but is more difficult to diagnose with an insidious course over a number of weeks. The introduction of zidovudine, which is toxic to bone-marrow, has made the prophylactic use of other potentially marrow-suppressant drugs such as TMP/SMZ controversial, although no specific interactions between zidovudine and TMP/SMZ or Fansidar have been demonstrated.

References

Allegra, C. J., Chabner, B. A., Tuazon, C. U., Ogata-Arakaki, D., Baird, B., Drake, J. C., *et al.* (1987). Trimetrexate for the treatment of pneumocystis carinii pneumonia in patients with the acquired immune deficiency syndrome. *New England Journal of Medicine* **317**, 978–85.

Editorial (1986). *American Review of Respiratory Diseases* **133**, 513–4.

Erban, J. K. (1987). Letter. *Annals of Internal Medicine* **106**, 475.

Fischl, M. A., Richman, D. D., Grieco, M. H. Gottlieb, M. S., Volberding, P. A., Laskin, D. L., *et al.* (1987). The efficacy of azidothymidine (AZT) in the treatment of patients with AIDS and AIDS-related complex. *New England Journal of Medicine* **317**, 185–91.

Gazzard, B. G., Anderson, M. & Gardner, T. (1987). The importance of clinical and laboratory parameters in the management of AIDS pneumonias. *III International Congress on AIDS, Washington,* p. 333.

Gottlieb, M. S., Knight, S. Mitsuyasu, R., Weisman, J., Roth, M. & Young, L. S. (1984). Prophylaxis of PCP infection in AIDS with pyrimethamine sulphaoxine. *Lancet ii*, 398–9.

Gottlieb, M. S., Schroff, R., Shanker, H. M., Weisman, J. D., Fan, P. T., Wolf, R. A. *et al.* (1981). Pneumocystis carinii pneumonia and mucosal candidiasis in previously healthy homosexual men: evidence of a new acquired cellular deficiency. *New England Journal of Medicine* **305**, 1425–7.

Hollander, H. (1985). Leukopenia trimethoprim sulphamethoxazol and folinic acid. *Annals of Internal Medicine* **102**, 138.

Hughes, W. T., Kuhn, S., Chaudry, S., Feldman, S., Verzosa, M. & Aur, R. J. A. (1977). Successful chemoprophylaxis of pneumocystis carnii pneumonitis. *New England Journal of Medicine* **297**, 1419–27.

Ivady, G. & Paldy, H. (1958). A new form of treatment of interstitial plasma cell pneumonia in premature infants with pentavalent antimony and aromatic diamines. *Monatsschrift Für Kinderheilkunde* **106**, 10–4.

Kinzie, B. J. & Taylor, J. W. (1984). Trimethoprim and folinic acid. *Annals of Internal Medicine* **101**, 565.

Kovacs, J. A., Hiemenz, J. W., Macher, A. M., Stover, D., Murray, H. W., Shelhamer, J. *et al.* (1984). Pneumocystis carinii pneumonia a comparison between patients with the acquired immune deficiency syndrome and patients with other immunodeficiences. *Annals of Internal Medicine* **100**, 663–71.

Leoung, G. S., Mills, J., Hopewell, P. C., Hughes, W. & Wofsy, C. (1986). Dapsone-trimethoprim and pneumocystis carinii pneumonia in the acquired immunodeficiency syndrome. *Annals of Internal Medicine* **105**, 45–8.

McFadden, D. K., Hyland, R. H., Inouye, T., Edelson, J. D., Rodrigues, C. H. & Rebuck, A. S. (1987). Corticosteroids as adjunctive therapy in treatment of pneumocystis carinii pneumonia in patients with the acquired immune deficiency syndrome *Lancet i*, 1477–9.

McLees, B. D., Barlow, J. L. R., Kuzma, R. J., Baringtang, D. C. & Schecter, P. R. (1987). Studies on successful eflornithine treatment of pneumocystis carinii pneumonia (PCP) in AIDS patients failing conventional therapy. *Third International Congress on AIDS, Washington*, p. 155.

Medina, I., Leoung, G. S., Mills, J., Hopewell, P., Feigel, D. & Wofsy, C. (1987). Oral therapy in Pneumocystis carinii pneumonia (PCP) in AIDS. A randomized double-blind trial of trimethoprim and sulphamethoxazole (S) versus dapsone trimethoprim for first episode pneumocystis carinii pneumonia in AIDS. *Third International Congress on AIDS, Washington*, p. 208.

Montgomery, B. A., Luce, J. M., Turner, J., Lin, E. T., Debs, R. J., Corkery, K. J. *et al.* (1987). Aerosolised pentamidine as sole therapy in pneumocystis carinii pneumonia in patients with the acquired immunodeficiency syndrome. *Lancet ii*, 480–3.

Mottin, D., Denis, M., Dombret, H., Rossert, J., Mayaud, C. H. & Akoun, G. (1987). Role for steroids in treatment of Pneumocystis carinii pneumonia in AIDS. *Lancet ii*, 519.

Navin, T. R., Miller, K. D., Satriale, R. F. & Lobel, H. O. (1985). Adverse reactions associated with pyrimethamine/sulphadoxine prophylaxis in pneumocystis carinii infections of AIDS. *Lancet i*, 332.

Pozniak, A. L., Tung, K. T., Swinburn, C. R., Tovey, S., Semple, S. J. G. & Johnson, N. McI. (1986). Clinical and bronchoscopic diagnosis of suspected pneumonia related to AIDS. *British Medical Journal* **293**, 797–9.

Rosen, M. J., Einstein, T., Chuang, M. & Brown, L. K. (1983). Response to therapy of pneumocystis carinii pneumonia in patients with the acquired immunodeficiency syndrome. *Chest* **84**, 347.

Tuazon, C. U. & Labriola, A. M. (1987). Management of infectious and immunological complications of acquired immunodeficiency syndrome (AIDS) current and future prospects. *Drugs* **33**, 66–84.

Western, K. A., Perera, D. R. & Schultz, M. G. (1970). Pentamidine isethionate in the treatment of pneumocystis carinii pneumonia. *Annals of Internal Medicine* **73**, 695–702.

Wharton, J. M., Coleman, D. L., Wofsy, C. B., Lace, J. M., Blumenfield, W. & Hadley, I. C., *et al.* (1986). Trimethoprim-sulphamethoxazole or pentamidine for pneumocystis carinii pneumonia in the acquired immunodeficiency syndrome. *Annals of Internal Medicine* **105**, 37–44.

Winston, D. J., Law, W. K., Gale, R. P. & Young, L. S. Trimethoprim sulphamethoxazole for the treatment of pneumocystis carinii pneumonia. (1980). *Annals of Internal Medicine* **92**, 762–9.

Wofsy, C. B. (1987). Use of trimethoprim-sulphamethoxazole in the treatment of pneumocystis carinii pneumonitis in patients with acquired immune deficiency syndrome. *Review of Infectious Diseases* **9**, *Suppl. 2*, S184–94.

Journal of Antimicrobial Chemotherapy (1989) **23**, *Suppl. A*, 77–82

Toxoplasmosis in AIDS patients

Carmelita U. Tuazon

*Division of Infectious Diseases, Department of Medicine,
George Washington University Medical Center,
2150 Pennsylvania Avenue, NW Washington, DC 20037, USA*

In patients with AIDS, toxoplasmosis is the most common cause of CNS mass lesions. Diagnosis is made on the basis of clinical presentation and CAT scan findings and confirmed by demonstration of tachyzoites and/or cysts in tissues obtained by needle aspiration or brain biopsy. Response to therapy with pyrimethamine and sulphadiazine is usually prompt but therapy has to be continued for the lifetime of AIDS patients with CNS toxoplasmosis. To date, no alternative regimens of single or combination drugs appear to be effective in patients who fail, or are unable to tolerate pyrimethamine and sulphadiazine therapy. Relapse rate is high. Clearly, there is a need to organize prospective controlled studies to assess the role of agents such as clindamycin, trimetrexate and other drugs in the treatment of CNS toxoplasmosis in patients with AIDS.

Introduction

There is a wide spectrum of central nervous system (CNS) complications seen in the AIDS population. In a comprehensive review of 315 patients, nonviral infections comprised 51% of cases, viral infections about 33%, neoplastic processes 10%, and the remaining 10% were attributed to cerebrovascular complications, multiple intracranial pathologies and miscellaneous cases (Levy, Bredesen & Rosenblum, 1985). Of the 162 nonviral infections, toxoplasmosis comprised about two thirds of cases.

Before recognition of AIDS, central nervous system (CNS) toxoplasmosis was a rare entity even in the setting of immunosuppression. In the 1980s CNS toxoplasmosis is one of the most common opportunistic infections seen in patients with AIDS and ranks as the leading cause of CNS mass lesions.

The incidence of CNS toxoplasmosis has been estimated to range between 3% and 40% of patients with AIDS. Projections however, have been as high as 20,000 to 40,000 cases of CNS toxoplasmosis in the USA by 1991 (Luft & Remington, 1988).

As has been previously noted, it may be difficult to make a definitive diagnosis of toxoplasmosis as the cause of focal encephalitis in the AIDS population (Krick & Remington, 1978). A wide variety of infectious and neoplastic processes singly or in combination have been reported to cause inflammatory central nervous system lesions. Fungal pathogens such as *Aspergillus*, *Candida* and *Cryptococcus* spp.; viruses, e.g. cytomegalovirus (CMV) and herpes simplex; typical and atypical mycobacteria; atypical malignancies e.g. Kaposi's sarcoma and lymphoma; and human immunodeficiency virus (HIV) infections have all been implicated as aetiologies of CNS lesions (Levy *et al.*, 1985; Snow & Lavyne, 1985).

77

Clinical diagnosis

Diagnosis of toxoplasma encephalitis may be suspected on clinical grounds. Of those showing abnormalities, the most frequent are neurological which may be focal or general (Wanke et al., 1987; Leport et al., 1988). Seizures have been reported in about 40% of cases and focal neurological abnormalities in 30% to 50% of patients with CNS toxoplasmosis. Focal neurological abnormalities include hemiparesis, hemiplegia, hemisensory loss, cranial nerve palsies, aphasia, ataxia and alexia. Meningeal symptoms have been reported in 11% of cases. Confusion, coma and psychosis have been observed in 10% to 30% of patients. Fever, although a nonspecific symptom, is present in 55%–75% of patients with CNS toxoplasmosis (Table I). Cerebrospinal fluid analysis may show signs of inflammation in some patients but is usually not helpful in making the diagnosis (Wanke et al., 1987).

Radiology

Computerized axial tomography (CAT) has been extremely valuable in diagnosing CNS toxoplasmosis. The density of lesions and the contrast enhancement of CNS toxoplasmosis lesions has shown substantial variability. Contrast enhancement of the lesions has been reported in 80% to 97% of cases (Wanke et al., 1987; Leport et al., 1988). Lesions have been reported as solitary or multiple and isodense or hypodense. The location of lesions has been variable but the majority of the masses are noted in cerebral hemispheres and basal ganglia. Mild to severe oedema is present on CAT scan in almost all patients. In patients with a clinical presentation compatible with CNS toxoplasmosis, in whom lesions are not detected by CAT scan, magnetic resonance imaging (MRI) may be helpful (Levy et al., 1985).

Serology

Although the majority of patients with CNS toxoplasmosis undergo serological investigation, a useful diagnostic method has not emerged. IgM antibodies are usually not present. Although IgG antibodies are predictably positive, this finding has been reported in 40% to 50% of healthy individuals in the US with chronic, inactive infection. In France, approximately 80% of the general population has evidence of previous infection. In a recent study IgM antibody to *Toxoplasma gondii* has been demonstrated in as many as 20% of patients with AIDS and CNS toxoplasmosis (Luft & Remington, 1988). In some patients, increase of antibodies in the CSF may be helpful in making the diagnosis. Twenty-three of 37 patients with AIDS and CNS toxoplasmosis had detectable titres in the CSF (Potasman et al., 1988). Sixteen of the 23 patients were evaluated for intrathecal production of antibody to *T. gondii* and 11 were positive. This was demonstrated in patients with IgG antibody titres of 1 : 128 to 1 : 4096. The authors suggest that local antibody production may depend on the proximity of the encephalitic process to the meninges. Antigen detection has not been proven to be useful for the diagnosis of CNS toxoplasmosis. Western blot analysis has been used to determine if antibodies recognizing specific toxoplasma antigens could be detected in AIDS patients with toxoplasma encephalitis. A wide diversity of antibody response among patients studies was observed which may represent antigenic diversity of toxoplasma strains (Weiss et al., 1988a).

Table I. Clinical presentation of AIDS patients with CNS toxoplasmosis

	Wanke et al. (1987) No. (%)	Leport et al. (1988) No. (%)
No. of patients evaluated	14	35
Neurological		
seizures	6 (43)	14 (40)
focal neurological signs	4 (30)	17 (49)
mental status change	2 (14)	
coma		8 (23)
confusion		11 (31)
meningeal symptoms		4 (11)
psychosis	1 (7)	
anaemia	1 (7)	
Fever	8 (57)	26 (74)

Table II. Adverse reactions to treatment of CNS toxoplasmosis

	Wanke et al. (1987)	Leport et al. (1988)
Incidence of toxicity	7/13 (54%)	25/35 (71%)
Haematological		
neutropenia	4/7 (57%)	17/35 (61%)
thrombocytopenia		13/35 (32%)
Fever	3/7 (43%)	
Rash	2/7 (30%)	12/35 (45%)
Liver function abnormalities		2/35 (6%)

Microbiology

Direct examination for parasites of Wright-Giemsa stained smears of brain aspirate or other tissue specimens, or centrifuged sediment of cerebrospinal fluid (CSF) may be diagnostic. However positive identifications are quite low and additional specimens derived from mouse inoculation and tissue culture techniques may also be helpful.

A definitive diagnosis can be made from brain biopsy with demonstration of the organisms. If needle biopsy or aspiration is the only feasible biopsy technique careful guidance by stereotaxis is highly desirable. In addition to the lack of sensitivity and specificity of using the needle biopsy technique sampling errors may occur. The atypical cellular response seen histologically may be difficult to distinguish from lymphoma.

Because of technical difficulties arising from the anatomical location of the mass lesion, and a phobia of AIDS of some neurosurgeons, the diagnosis of CNS toxoplasmosis by brain biopsy has been controversial. It has been recommended and is accepted general practice that AIDS patients with CNS mass lesions are presumed to have toxoplasmosis and treated as such. In the setting of technical difficulty due to the anatomical location, or in a population of patients who do not have a predisposition to other opportunistic infections a therapeutic trial with pyrimethamine and sulphadiazine seems a reasonable alternative. A clinical and radiological response may be expected within seven to ten days of initiation of therapy. However, one should keep in mind that in certain subgroups such as Haitians, Africans and intravenous drug abusers, tuberculosis is an important diagnosis. Other pathogens, e.g. *Cryptococcus*, *Mycobacterium tuberculosis* and *Aspergillus* spp., or malignancy coexisting with *T. gondii* have been reported (Levy *et al.*, 1985).

Therapy

The combination of pyrimethamine and sulphadiazine has been shown to be the most efficacious regimen in the treatment of patients with AIDS and toxoplasmosis (Wong *et al.*, 1984; Wanke *et al.*, 1987; Leport *et al.*, 1988). The two drugs act synergistically by sequential blockade of folic acid metabolism. The activity is limited to the replicating tachyzoite, and the cyst form remains a viable source of organism able to rupture and reinitiate the process. Such a latent process probably accounts for the very high incidence of relapses among AIDS patients.

The serum and CSF levels of pyrimethamine and sulphadiazine necessary for inhibiting or killing *T. gondii* have not been established. There are minimal data available on concentrations of pyrimethamine in the serum and CSF. After oral administration of 25 and 50 mg doses of pyrimethamine, CSF levels ranging from 101 to 246 ng/ml and 417 to 463 ng/ml have been obtained, respectively. The CSF concentration is about 12·7–26·5% of that achieved in serum (Weiss *et al.*, 1988*a*). Serum concentrations of 260–1411 ng/ml after 25 mg of pyrimethamine and 1333 to 4472 ng/ml after 50 mg of pyrimethamine have been detected.

Most recently in-vitro testing has demonstrated that pyrimethamine has good in-vitro activity and is synergistic with sulphadiazine. Pyrimethamine concentrations of 0·5 to 1·0 mg/l achieved the same effect as pyrimethamine at 0·1 mg/l combined with sulphadiazine at 25 mg/l (Harris *et al.*, 1988).

To date, no effective alternative therapeutic regimen has been reported for patients who do not respond to or are unable to tolerate pyrimethamine and sulphadiazine. In-vitro studies have demonstrated that clindamycin alone or in combination with sulphadiazine has no significant effect. In animal studies, high doses of clindamycin have been shown to be efficacious. However, no eradication of organisms from the brain was observed. Recently, clindamycin has been shown to decrease mortality in mice injected intracerebrally with *T. gondii* (Hofflin & Remington, 1987).

Other drugs tested *in vitro* include spiramycin, difluoromethylornithine (DFMO) and methotrexate all of which were not effective. Of note was the toxoplasmicidal activity of 5-fluorocytosine at doses ten-fold lower than that used for cancer chemotherapy (Harris *et al.*, 1988).

A new drug, trimetrexate, used in the treatment of cancer has been tested, both *in vitro* and *in vivo*. Trimetrexate is a lipid soluble antifolate that has been demonstrated to have high activity in inhibiting the dihydrofolate reductase of *T. gondii* (Kovacs *et al.*, 1987). The drug is also taken up rapidly by *T. gondii* tachyzoites. The structural modification of trimetrexate, which is more lipid soluble than methotrexate, may account for the enhanced antiprotozoan effect. *In vitro*, at a dose of 10^{-7} M, trimetrexate completely inhibited *T. gondii* replication compared with 10^{-6} M pyrimethamine and 10^{-4} M trimethoprim. In-vitro and in-vivo studies suggest that trimetrexate alone, or combined with a sulphonamide, may provide a safe and effective alternative for pyrimethamine plus sulphonamide for the treatment of toxoplasmosis.

Also tested in the same system was sulphadiazine which, at levels of 100–200 mg/l, had no effect on in-vitro *T. gondii* replication. Greater inhibition was demonstrated when sulphadiazine was combined with DHFR inhibitors.

In mouse studies, pyrimethamine alone appeared to be more effective than trimetrexate alone. This finding may be related to the half-life of the drugs. The pyrimethamine $t_{\frac{1}{2}}$ is about 6 h while the trimetrexate $t_{\frac{1}{2}}$ is only about 50 min. The $t_{\frac{1}{2}}$ of pyrimethamine and trimetrexate in humans is 96 and 9·5 h, respectively. It appears however, that trimetrexate penetrates the CNS and this is important in the treatment of patients with cerebral disease who require long term therapy.

In clinical studies, pyrimethamine and sulphadiazine are efficacious in the treatment of AIDS patients with CNS toxoplasmosis. The major problem in the treatment of CNS toxoplasmosis, similar to the other opportunistic infections seen in patients with AIDS, is the very high relapse rate. Daily therapy for documented disease should be continued for the lifetime of patients with AIDS.

Our clinical experience with combination therapy with pyrimethamine and sulphadiazine demonstrated clinical and radiological improvement in 11 of 13 patients studied (Wanke *et al.*, 1987). A decrease in size of the lesion in eight of ten patients was noted on CAT scan. Two of the 13 patients did not demonstrate clinical or radiological benefit from sulphadiazine and pyrimethamine despite 30 and 56 days of therapy. Toxicity occurred in seven of 13 patients, manifested as neutropenia, fever and rash (Table II). Recrudescence occurred when combination therapy was discontinued, despite six months of therapy in one patient. Autopsies performed in five patients showed evidence of *T. gondii* except in one case who had evidence of invasive candidiasis at the biopsy site.

A more recent report on the experience with 35 patients with AIDS and CNS toxoplasmosis confirmed earlier observations regarding outcome of therapy (Leport *et al.*, 1988). In this series, the mean duration of total therapy was six months. Efficacy of the regimen was observed in 31/35 (89%) with complete resolution in 10/35 (29%) and partial improvement in 21 (60%). Failure was noted in 4/35 (11%) of patients treated for a mean duration of five weeks. Treatment was administered promptly with the mean time from the onset of neurological signs to the initiation of therapy being ten days (range 1–70 days). Six patients experienced ten relapses which occurred within six weeks of discontinuation of therapy in seven of ten. Retreatment with the combination led to complete resolution of the relapse in eight cases.

In this study, 24 patients were evaluable for the efficacy of long term therapy. Fourteen of 24 (58%) achieved complete resolution and ten had late clinical and/or CAT scan sequelae.

In patients who died and had autopsies performed, brain specimens demonstrated histopathological evidence of acute toxoplasmosis with multiple foci of necrosis, and extensive inflammation with multiple cysts in 3/15 (20%) of patients. In the remaining 80% less active or quiescent CNS *T. gondii* infection was noted with absent or few foci of necrosis and few cysts or calcifications.

In addition to the high relapse rate, another major problem in the treatment of CNS toxoplasmosis is the high frequency of adverse reactions as observed in all the reported series. Seventy one per cent of patients developed side effects in this study (Leport *et al.,* 1988). Haematological toxicity was common, manifested as leucopenia and thrombocytopenia, and was observed in 61% and 32% of cases, respectively. A rash was noted in 45% of patients treated, and liver function abnormalities in less than 10% of cases. The therapeutic regimens were altered in about a third of cases because of drug toxicity (Table II).

Though drug toxicity induced by pyrimethamine and/or sulphadiazine and treatment failures are undesirable, alternative therapeutic regimens are limited. Although clindamycin has been demonstrated to be effective in animal studies, there is minimal experience with the use of this drug in the treatment of CNS toxoplasmosis in AIDS patients.

Clinical experience with the use of trimetrexate in patients with CNS toxoplasmosis and AIDS is also limited. To date, nine patients were treated at the National Institute of Health and George Washington University Medical Center and five patients responded for a period ranging from two weeks to three months. One patient remained stable for three months and three patients showed no response.

References

Harris, C., Salgo, M. P., Tanowitz, H. & Wittner, M. (1988). In-vitro assessment of antimicrobials against *Toxoplasma gondii*. *Journal of Infectious Diseases* **157**, 14–22.

Hofflin, J. M. & Remington, J. S. (1987). Clindamycin in a murine model of toxoplasmic encephalitis. *Antimicrobial Agents and Chemotherapy* **31**, 492–6.

Kovacs, J. A., Allegra, C. J., Chabner, B. A., Swan, J. C., Drake, J., Lunde, M. *et al.* (1987). Potent effect of trimetrexate, a lipid-soluble antifolate, on *Toxoplasma gondii*. *Journal of Infectious Diseases* **155**, 1027–32.

Krick, M. A. & Remington, J. S. (1978). Current concepts in parasitology: toxoplasmosis in the adult—an overview. *New England Journal of Medicine* **298**, 550–3.

Leport, C., Raffi, F., Matheron, S., Katlama, C., Regnier, B., Saimot, A. G. *et al.* (1988). Treatment of central nervous system toxoplasmosis with pyrimethamine/sulfadiazine combination in 35 patients with the acquired immunodeficiency syndrome. *American Journal of Medicine* **84**, 94–100.

Levy, R. M., Bredesen, D. E. & Rosenblum, M. (1985). Neurologic manifestations of the acquired immunodeficiency syndrome (AIDS): experience of UCSF and review of literature. *Journal of Neurosurgery* **62**, 475–95.

Luft, B. J. & Remington, J. S. (1988). Toxoplasmic encephalitis. *Journal of Infectious Diseases* **157**, 1–6.

Potasman, I., Resnick, L., Luft, B. J. & Remington, J. S. (1988). Intrathecal production of antibodies against *Toxoplasma gondii* in patients with toxoplasmic encephalitis and the acquired immunodeficiency syndrome (AIDS). *Annals of Internal Medicine* **108**, 49–51.

Snow, R. B. & Lavyne, M. H. (1985). Intracranial space occupying lesions in acquired immune deficiency syndrome patients . *Neurosurgery* **16**, 148–53.

Wanke, C., Tuazon, C. U., Kovacs, A., Dina, T., Davis, D. O., Barton, N. *et al.* (1987). Toxoplasma encephalitis in patients with acquired immune deficiency syndrome: diagnosis and response to therapy. *American Journal of Tropical Medicine and Hygiene* **36**, 509–16.

Weiss, L. M., Harris, C., Berger, M., Tanowitz, A. B. & Wittner, M. (1988*a*). Pyrimethamine concentrations in serum and cerebrospinal fluid during treatment of acute toxoplasma encephalitis in patients with AIDS. *Journal of Infectious Diseases* **154**, 580–3.

Weiss, L. M., Udem, S. A., Tanowitz, H. & Wittner, M. (1988*b*). Western Blot analysis of the antibody response of patients with AIDS and toxoplasma encephalitis: antigenic diversity among *Toxoplasma* strains. *Journal of Infectious Diseases* **157**, 7–13.

Wong, B., Gold, W. M., Brown, A., Lange, M., Fried, R., Grieco, M. *et al.* (1984). Central nervous system toxoplasmosis in homosexual men and parenteral drug abusers. *Annals of Internal Medicine* **100**, 36–42.

Journal of Antimicrobial Chemotherapy (1989) **23**, *Suppl. A*, 83–87

Diagnosis and management of HIV-infected patients with diarrhoea

J. Louise Gerberding

Department of Medicine, University of California, San Francisco and Medical Service, San Francisco General Hospital, 1001 Potrero Avenue, San Francisco, CA 94110, USA

Diarrhoea and weight loss are found in more than 50% of patients with AIDS and in some patients can be so severe that death may occur even in the absence of opportunistic infections. Systematic evaluation of diarrhoeal illness in HIV-infected patients will often identify a treatable aetiology. Despite the tendency for recurrences, the majority of patients will respond to anti-infective therapy. A practical approach to the diagnosis and management of HIV-infected patients with diarrhoea is presented in this article.

Introduction

The gastrointestinal tract is a common target organ system in patients infected with human immunodeficiency virus (HIV). Diarrhoea and weight loss are found in more than 50% of patients with AIDS and are also frequently present in those with less severe clinical manifestations of immunodeficiency (Cone *et al.*, 1986; Santangelo & Krejs, 1986; Cello, 1988; Laughon *et al.*, 1988; Smith *et al.*, 1988). In some patients, these symptoms and associated malabsorption are so severe that death may occur even in the absence of opportunistic infection.

Diagnosis and management

Diagnosing the specific aetiology of diarrhoeal illness in HIV-infected patients is challenging because of the variety of infectious as well as neoplastic and inflammatory processes which may produce identical symptoms (Table I). As with other clinical syndromes in AIDS, the approach to the patient with diarrhoeal illness is oriented toward diagnosing treatable aetiologies and avoiding unnecessary invasive procedures.

Localization of infection to either the small bowel or the colon can help to suggest likely pathogens and direct the diagnostic process. Cramping periumbilical pain associated with large volume diarrhoea and weight loss suggest small bowel enteritis. With colorectal involvement, diarrhoea is usually smaller in volume and associated with tenesmus and left lower quadrant pain. Stools may contain small amounts of bright red blood. When symptoms are accompanied by proctalgia and dyskesia, proctitis should be considered (Cello, 1988).

0305–7453/89/23A083 + 05 $02.00/0

Table I. Infectious aetiologies of diarrhoea and malabsorption in AIDS

Bacteria	Protozoa	Viruses
Salmonella spp.	*Cryptosporidium*	HIV
Shigella spp.	*I. belli*	
Campylobacter spp.	*G. lamblia*	cytomegalovirus
M. avium-intracellulare	*E. histolytica*	herpes simplex virus

Stool cultures

Stool samples should be obtained from all patients with diarrhoea, examined for faecal leucocytes, and cultured for salmonella, shigella, and campylobacter. Blood cultures should be obtained in patients with fever or other constitutional symptoms, since bacteraemia in association with enteric infection is more common in AIDS and ARC patients than in other patient populations (Celum *et al.*, 1987).

Antimicrobial treatment of diagnosed enteric bacterial pathogens in HIV-infected patients is indicated. Parenteral therapy is usually recommended for the initial management of bacteraemic patients. The vast majority will have a favourable symptomatic and microbiological response to treatment. Unfortunately, drug toxicity is a frequent occurrence, particularly when ampicillin or trimethoprim-sulphamethoxazole are administered. In addition, relapses and recurrences are common, even after prolonged treatment. Recurrent infections are often complicated by the emergence of resistant organisms (Glaser *et al.*, 1985; Profeta *et al.*, 1985; Dworkin *et al.*, 1986; Perlman *et al.*, 1988). In our experience, the new quinolones appear to be promising for the treatment of salmonella, shigella, and campylobacter enteritis in AIDS and ARC patients. In a small series of patients with enteric infections, refractory or resistant to conventional antimicrobials, treated with ciprofloxacin at San Francisco General Hospital, clinical response was excellent, no drug toxicity was apparent, and chronic suppressive therapy was effective and well-tolerated.

Evaluation for protozoal infections

At least three stool specimens should be examined to identify ova or parasites. A saline wet preparation of fresh liquid stool may demonstrate trophozoites of *Entamoeba histolytica* or *Giardia lamblia*. Stool preserved in formalin or polyvinyl alcohol and stained with iron haematoxylin or trichrome often demonstrates the cysts of these organisms and can be used with formed stool where trophozoites are rarely detected. Conventional therapeutic regimens are adequate to treat these infections even in AIDS patients. Surprisingly, extraintestinal ameobiasis is distinctly uncommon in AIDS.

Cryptosporidium is one of the most common pathogens isolated from AIDS patients with diarrhoea (Laughon *et al.*, 1988). Modified acid-fast stains for *Cryptosporidium* oocytes should be performed on stools from all symptomatic patients. Concentration techniques may be helpful in identifying the presence of cysts in patients with formed stools (Soave & Armstrong, 1986). Cryptosporidiosis in AIDS patients is persistent and may be severe or even fatal if malabsorption and cachexia ensue. Numerous chemotherapeutic agents including metronidazole, quinidine-clindamycin, and pentamidine have been tried in an attempt to eradicate or suppress the symptoms of cryptosporidiosis but have met with little success (Soave & Armstrong, 1986). Spiramycin, a macrolide antibiotic, has been useful in a subset of patients and is relatively non-toxic (Pilla, Ryback & Chandrasekar, 1987). To date, there is no proven effective therapy although a variety of investigational agents are currently undergoing evaluation. The importance of supportive care directed towards decreasing intestinal motility, maintaining fluid and electrolyte balance, and parenteral feeding should not be overlooked.

Isospora belli produces symptoms identical to *Cryptosporidium*. Stool specimens often reveal Charcot–Leyden crystals with isosporiasis. Since oocytes may be shed intermittently, multiple specimens should be obtained and concentrated before evaluation. Trimethoprim-sulphamethoxazole is effective in eliminating symptoms in the majority of patients and has been used successfully to treat recurrences (DeHovitz et al., 1986). Chronic suppressive therapy with trimethoprim-sulphamethoxazole or weekly pyrimethamine-sulfadoxine is recommended to prevent recurrent infection, which occurs in more than 40% of cases (DeHovitz et al., 1986).

Proctosigmoidoscopy

Endoscopic evaluation is indicated in all symptomatic patients with diarrhoea when the above investigations fail to identify an aetiology or when symptoms of proctocolitis are present. Cytomegalovirus infection produces shallow ulceration of the mucosa accompanied by submucosal haemorrhages. Directed biopsies should be obtained for histopathological evaluation and culture. The value of ganciclovir for the treatment of cytomegalovirus colitis has not been definitively established, but anecdotal reports suggest that at least some patients may respond (Chachoua et al., 1987; Jacobson & Mills, 1988).

Herpes simplex virus is the cause in a large proportion of patients with proctitis and ulceration, and can be readily diagnosed by directed biopsy. Parenteral therapy with acyclovir is usually efficacious, but the infection may recur. Chlamydia and neisseria cultures should also be performed since these organisms are not unusual in homosexual patients with persistent diarrhoea. Biopsies should be performed even in the absence of focal pathology to exclude *Cryptosporidium* in the rare case where stool examination has failed to demonstrate the organism (Cello, 1988).

Kaposi's sarcoma, carcinomas, lymphoma, and idiopathic inflammatory bowel disease produce clinical syndromes indistinguishable from infectious diarrhoea in HIV-infected patients. Proctosigmoidoscopy is extremely valuable in diagnosing these disorders and is therefore routinely recommended when an infectious aetiology has not been established.

Pseudomembranous enterocolitis should be considered in patients with diarrhoea following antibacterial treatment. Histological examination of pseudomembrane biopsies from the distal colon and detection of *Clostridium difficile* toxin confirm the diagnosis. Oral treatment with vancomycin or metronidazole is usually effective. A trial of parenteral metronidazole in patients with extremely rapid intestinal transit times who fail with oral regimens may be of benefit.

Small bowel biopsy

Small bowel biopsy is indicated when stool samples and lower intestinal endoscopy fail to reveal a diagnosis. Multiple biopsies can be obtained with either oral capsule techniques or fibreoptic endoscopy. Endoscopy has the advantage of allowing inspection of the oesophagus and stomach in patients with symptoms referable to these sites (Cello, 1988).

Cytomegalovirus ulceration and vasculitis is easily diagnosed from histopathological study of biopsy specimens. Cytomegalovirus should not be considered the cause on the basis of a positive culture in the absence of focal pathology since this organism is ubiquitous in AIDS patients. In a minority of patients, cytomegalovirus ulcerations may result in intestinal perforation.

Mycobacterium avium–intracellulare (MAI) is presumptively diagnosed by the presence of PAS-positive macrophages in biopsy specimens and is confirmed by culture. MAI can be distinguished from Whipple's disease by acid-fast staining (Roth *et al.*, 1985). The indications for treating MAI remain controversial since there is currently no evidence that treatment with any regimen alters the course of the infection or improves long-term outcome.

Recent studies suggest that HIV may directly invade the small bowel and produce recognizable pathological changes. In-situ hybridization of biopsy specimens from the duodenum have revealed HIV-infected cells in the lamina propria (Nelson *et al.*, 1988). Intracellular virus-like particles, lymphocytic infiltrates, non-specific inflammatory changes, and villous atrophy have also been observed (McLoughlin *et al.*, 1987; Cello, 1988). The detection of HIV RNA in enterochromaffin cells has led to the hypothesis that HIV infection could be directly responsible for neurogenic diarrhoea by stimulating the production of neuropeptides (Nelson *et al.*, 1988). The response of idiopathic or other forms of diarrhoeal illness to zidovudine and other antiviral agents has not yet been systematically studied.

Defective mucosal immunity and bacterial overgrowth has been suggested as a contributing factor to diarrhoea in AIDS patients (Budhraja *et al.*, 1987). Analysis of lymphocyte subpopulations from duodenal biopsies have demonstrated a reduction of T-helper lymphocytes and a reversal of the T-helper/T-suppressor ratio which correlated with the presence of bacterial colonization. The benefit of empirical broad spectrum antibacterial therapy for these patients has not yet been determined.

Summary

Systematic evaluation of diarrhoea in HIV-infected patients will often identify a treatable cause. Despite the tendency for recurrences, the majority of patients will respond to anti-infective therapy. Hopefully, the development of successful drugs for HIV and cryptosporidiosis will reduce the impact of diarrhoeal illness in this patient population.

References

Budhraja, M., Levendoglu, H., Kocka, F. Mangkornkanok, M. & Sherer, R. (1987 Duodenal mucosal T-cell subpopulation and bacterial cultures in acquired immune deficiency syndrome. *Americal Journal of Gastroenterology* **82,** 427–31.

Cello, J. P. (1988). Gastrointestinal manifestations of HIV infection. In *Infectious Disease Clinics of North America*. Vol. 2 (2) (Sande, M. A. & Volberding, P. V., Eds), pp. 387–96. W. B. Saunders, Philadelphia.

Celum, C. L., Chaisson, R. E., Rutherford, G. W., Barnhart, J. L. & Echenberg, D. F. (1987) Incidence of salmonellosis in patients with AIDS. *Journal of Infectious Diseases* **156,** 998–1002.

Chachoua, A., Dieterich, D., Krasinski, K., Greene, J., Laubenstein, L., Wernz, J. *et al.* (1987). 9-(1,3-Dihydroxy-2-propoxymethyl) guanine (ganciclovir) in the treatment of cytomegalovirus gastrointestinal disease with the acquired immunodeficiency syndrome. *Annals of Internal Medicine* **107,** 133–7.

Cone, L. A., Woodard, D. R., Potts, B. E., Byrd R. G., Alexander, R. M. & Last, M. D. (1986). An update on the acquired immunodeficiency syndrome (AIDS). Associated disorders of the alimentary tract. *Diseases of the Colon and Rectum* **29,** 60–4.

DeHovitz, J. A., Pape, J. W., Boncy, M. & Johnson, W. D. (1986). Clinical manifestations and therapy of *Isospora belli* infection in patients with the acquired immunodeficiency syndrome. *New England Journal of Medicine* **315,** 87–90.

Dworkin, B., Wormser, G. P., Abdoo, R. A., Cabello, F., Aguero, M. E. & Sivak, S. L. (1986). Persistence of multiply antibiotic-resistant *Campylobacter jejuni* in a patient with the acquired immune deficiency syndrome. *American Journal of Medicine* **80,** 965–70.

Glaser, J. B., Morton-Kute, L., Berger, S. R., Weber, J., Siegal, F. P., Lopez, C. *et al.* (1985). Recurrent *Salmonella typhimurium* bacteremia associated with the acquired immunodeficiency syndrome. *Annals of Internal Medicine* **102,** 189–93.

Jacobson, M. A. & Mills, J. (1988). Serious cytomegalovirus disease in the acquired immunodeficiency syndrome (AIDS). Clinical findings, diagnosis, and treatment. *Annals of Internal Medicine* **108,** 585–94.

Laughon, B. E., Druckman, D. A., Vernon, A., Quinn, T. C., Polk, B. F., Modlin, J. F. *et al.* (1988). Prevalence of enteric pathogens in homosexual men with and without acquired immunodeficiency syndrome. *Gastroenterology* **94,** 984–93.

McLoughlin, L. C., Nord, K. S., Joshi, V. V., Oleske, J. M. (1987). Severe gastrointestinal involvement in children with the acquired immunodeficiency syndrome. *Journal of Pediatric Gastroenterology and Nutrition* **6,** 517–24.

Nelson, J. A., Wiley, C. A., Reynolds-Kohler, C., Reese, C. E., Margaretten, W. & Levy, J. A. (1988). Human immunodeficiency virus detected in bowel epithelium from patients with gastrointestinal symptoms. *Lancet i,* 259–62.

Perlman, D. M., Ampel, N. M., Schifman, R. B., Cohn, D. L., Patton, C. M., Aguirre, M. L. *et al.* (1988). Persistent *Campylobacter jejuni* infections in patients infected with the human immunodeficiency virus (HIV). *Annals of Internal Medicine* **108,** 540–6.

Pilla, A. M., Rybak, M. J. & Chandrasekar, P. H. (1987). Spiramycin in the treatment of cryptosporidiosis. *Pharmacotherapy* **7,** 188–90.

Profeta, S., Forrester, C., Eng, R. H., Liu, R., Johnson, E., Palinkas, R. *et al.* (1985). *Salmonella* infections in patients with acquired immunodeficiency syndrome. *Archives of Internal Medicine* **145,** 670–2.

Roth, R. I., Owen, R. L., Keren, D. F. & Volberding, P. A. (1985). Intestinal infection with *Mycobacterium avium* in acquired immune deficiency syndrome (AIDS). Histological and clinical comparison with Whipple's disease. *Digestive Disease Science* **30,** 497–504.

Santangelo, W. C. & Krejs, G. J. (1986). Gastrointestinal manifestations of the acquired immunodeficiency syndrome. *American Journal of Medical Science* **292,** 328–34.

Smith, P. D., Lane, H. C., Gill, V. J., Manischewitz, J. F., Quinnan, G. V., Fauci, A. S. *et al.* (1988). Intestinal infections in patients with the acquired immunodeficiency syndrome (AIDS). Etiology and response to therapy. *Annals of Internal Medicine* **108,** 328–33.

Soave, R. & Armstrong, D. (1986). *Cryptosporidium* and cryptosporidiosis. *Reviews of Infectious Diseases* **8,** 1012–23.

Journal of Antimicrobial Chemotherapy (1989) **23**, *Suppl. A*, 89–105

Cytomegalovirus and the acquired immunodeficiency syndrome

A. S. Tyms[a]*, D. L. Taylor[b] and J. M. Parkin[c]

[a]*Departments of Medical Microbiology and* [c]*Immunology, St. Mary's Hospital Medical School, Paddington, London W2 IPG;* [b]*Division of Sexually Transmitted Diseases, Clinical Research Centre, Watford Road, Harrow, Middlesex HA1 3UJ, UK*

The acquired immunodeficiency syndrome (AIDS) is complex in nature with one major aetiological factor but with numerous other agents exploiting the immune incompetence. Cytomegaloviruses (CMV) form a little-defined group of viruses which naturally persist in man and respond readily to the relaxation in immune surveillance. A role for CMV and other herpesviruses in potentiating the underlying infection with human immune deficiency virus (HIV) cannot be totally excluded but CMV is well established as a major opportunist in AIDS. They are considered responsible for a range of diseases in AIDS patients including retinitis, gastrointestinal disease, pneumonitis and, less frequently, encephalitis. The pyrophosphate analogue foscarnet (phosphonoformate) and the deoxyguanosine analogue ganciclovir have both been used to treat CMV infections in AIDS patients. Results of uncontrolled studies have indicated efficacy with both drugs but the work with ganciclovir is particularly encouraging. This communication provides a review of CMV infections in AIDS patients with special reference to the experiences to-date in the use of ganciclovir and foscarnet.

Introduction

Human cytomegalovirus (CMV) is classified amongst the Herpesviridae and, like many of its counterparts, it is characterized by the ability to cause persistent or latent infections with potential for reactivation (Jordan, 1983). Infections with CMV are usually asymptomatic but in adults the virus can cause infectious mononucleosis, has serious consequences during pregnancy and results in major complications in immunocompromised individuals. Primary exposure to CMV or reactivation of endogenous virus in pregnancy can result in intrauterine infection causing a wide spectrum of disease in the newborn, including prematurity, mental retardation and sensory neural deafness (Stagno *et al.*, 1982; Peckham *et al.*, 1983). The incidence of CMV infection and disease after allogeneic transplantation of kidney, heart and liver is high (Betts, 1982) but infection with this virus is particularly devastating in bone-marrow transplant (BMT) recipients. Up to 20% of these patients contract serious disease, usually in the form of severe pneumonitis, with a fatality rate of about 80% (Meyers, Fleurnoy & Thomas, 1982).

CMV infection itself is known to be immunosuppressive (Rinaldo *et al.*, 1980; Carney *et al.*, 1981), and because of its frequent isolation from patients with AIDS the virus was suggested in the early 1980's to be a potential aetiological agent. Even

---

*Present address: Medical Research Council Collaborative Centre, 1–3 Burtonhole Lane, Mill Hill, London NW7 1AD, UK.

0305–7453/89/23A089 + 17 $02.00/0

though human immunodeficiency virus (HIV) is now considered to be the causative agent of AIDS, CMV infection is still of major importance owing to its ability to exploit the immune deficient state as an opportunist (Moskowitz *et al.*, 1985; Niedt & Schinella, 1985). CMV causes life-threatening and sight-threatening conditions in immunosuppressed patients and this demands effective antiviral chemotherapy, which may also help define the true role of CMV in AIDS.

The congener of acyclovir, 9(1,3-dihydroxypropoxymethyl)guanine (DHPG or ganciclovir) has been used to treat CMV infections in AIDS patients with major benefits in patient care (Collaborative DHPG Treatment Study Group, 1986; Chachoua *et al.*, 1987; Laskin *et al.*, 1987). Limited studies with the pyrophosphate analogue, phosphonoformic acid (foscarnet) have also demonstrated that this may be a clinically useful drug against CMV (Applerley *et al.*, 1985; Ringden *et al.*, 1985; Weber *et al.*, 1986).

Little is known about the natural history of CMV, its pathogenicity or strain variability. Furthermore, it is necessary to understand fully the mode of action of effective antiviral agents on virus growth both *in vitro* and *in vivo*. The present discussion of CMV in AIDS addresses some of the questions relating to disease, pathogenicity and treatment.

Incidence of CMV in AIDS patients and groups at risk for HIV infection

Groups at risk for HIV infection such as homosexual men and intravenous drug abusers, have high seroprevalence rates for CMV. It has become clear that venereal transmission is a prime factor in the spread of infection (Chretien, McGinniss & Muller, 1977; Handsfield *et al.*, 1985) and virus can be readily isolated from the cervix (Jordan *et al.*, 1973) and semen (Lang & Kummer, 1972; 1975). The latter association appears to be of major importance in transmission within homosexual groups. This is borne out by the high incidence of antibodies to CMV in homosexual men and the increased frequency of virus shedding (Drew *et al.*, 1981; Mintz *et al.*, 1983; Greenberg *et al.*, 1984). The frequency of antibody to CMV in homosexuals in three studies (Drew *et al.*, 1981; Mintz *et al.*, 1983; Greenberg *et al.*, 1984) was between 87–94%, almost twice that observed in heterosexuals. The isolation of infectious virus from these patients, in particular from the urine, also yielded significant differences between the two groups. Repeated exposure to high titres of CMV, particularly by anal-genital contact (Mintz *et al.*, 1983), must be considered a major means for CMV transmission.

Clinical manifestations of CMV infection in AIDS patients

In contrast to reactivation, primary infection with CMV is only rarely documented in patients with HIV infection. Of the cases that have been reported in patients with asymptomatic HIV infection or AIDS-related complex (ARC), overwhelming disease did not occur, but it appears that HIV infected individuals develop a mononucleosis type syndrome more frequently than the HIV negative population (Leport *et al.*, 1987).

CMV is frequently isolated from patients with HIV-infection in the absence of documented disease. For this reason, many centres require evidence of pathogenicity, such as the presence of inclusion bodies, or the growth of virus from tissue rather than body fluid, before a diagnosis of CMV-related disease is made. The correct diagnosis is

Table I. Cytomegalovirus-related disease in patients with AIDS

Site	Type of disease	Reference
Respiratory tract	Interstitial pneumonitis	Murray *et al.* (1984)
Nervous system	Encephalitis	Post *et al.* (1986)
	Retinitis	Friedman *et al.* (1983)
	Meningo-encephalitis	Edwards *et al.* (1985)
	Transverse myelitis	Jeantils *et al.* (1986)
	Subacute polyneuropathy	
Gastro-intestinal	Colitis/proctitis	Smith *et al.* (1988)
	Oesophageal/gastric/ duodenal inflammation/ulceration	Quinn (1987) Weber *et al.* (1986)
	Hepatitis	
	Acalcuric cholecystitis/ cholangitis	Saraux *et al.* (1987)
Adrenal gland	Necrosis, Addison's disease	Greene *et al.* (1984)
Vascular	Thrombosis syndromes	Bagley *et al.* (1986) Peterson & Stahl-Bayliss (1987)

of importance, as therapeutic agents having activity against CMV are undergoing trial with encouraging results. However, all agents used to date have side-effects and therefore must be used with caution. The advent of such drugs means that rapid diagnosis of CMV is essential and techniques such as DEAFF testing and dot-blot hybridization provide a useful addition to routine culture (Griffiths *et al.*, 1984).

Details of CMV-related disease in AIDS patients are summarized in Table I.

One of the most devastating diseases caused by CMV is retinitis (Friedman *et al.*, 1983) which is the only opportunist infection commonly to involve the eye. The earliest sign is the presence of granular white spots following a peri-vascular distribution. As the disease progresses haemorrhage and necrosis occur owing to infarction of retinal vessels. Without treatment the retinitis is progressive and blindness due to macular or optic nerve involvement may occur within weeks. Symptoms may predate fundoscopic signs by days or weeks and complaints of visual disturbances such as transient scotomas, 'floaters', or pain behind the eye are of potential importance. Cotton wool spots (CWS) are a well recognized feature of HIV infection and are a bad prognostic sign for the development of full-blown AIDS (Humphrey, Parkin & Marsh, 1986), but the cause of these is not certain. They tend to occur peri-vascularly and on histology are typical 'cytoid bodies' characteristic of microinfarction. Some studies using in-situ hybridization have demonstrated CMV in the retinae of patients with CWS (Kennedy *et al.*, 1986). Using the anti-CMV agent ganciclovir we have documented the resolution of typical CWS in patients with CMV disease at other sites and return of the lesions with relapse of disease suggesting that these may be CMV related (Parkin *et al.*, 1986). However, it is likely that there are many causes for CWS. They have been documented in 15% of cases of Pneumocystis carinii pneumonia without CMV infection (M. Helbert, personal communication) and pneumocystis has been found within the lesions. CWS may be a feature of immune complex deposition during episodes of opportunist infection or due to HIV-anti-HIV antibody interaction.

Cytomegalovirus has been associated with several diseases of the nervous system. The most common is a diffuse encephalitis or more rarely meningo-encephalitis (Post *et al.*, 1986; Edwards, Messing & McKendall, 1985). There are no particular distinguishing features of encephalitis caused by CMV.

The gastrointestinal tract is a common site of CMV disease. Primary infection with CMV, and some cases of reactivation, are accompanied by evidence of hepatitis due to infection of the liver. The emergence of CMV disease in patients with AIDS is generally associated with little or no change in liver function tests (LFT) although it is possible that the minor but persistent elevation of transaminases and alkaline phosphatase observed in many patients may be related to reactivation of CMV. The most common manifestation of CMV in the gastrointestinal tract is colitis. CMV disease in the gut is commonly associated with other opportunist infections or tumours. In a recent prospective study of 22 AIDS patients with diarrhoea nine patients were found to have CMV on biopsy. Five of the patients with CMV also had one or more additional infections, commonly atypical mycobacteria, salmonella, shigella, or campylobacter. However in four cases CMV was the only pathogen identified (Smith *et al.*, 1988). In the stomach and oesophagus CMV inclusion bodies have been documented within or around Kaposi sarcoma tissue (personal observation). Rarely CMV may invade the biliary tract causing acalcuric cholecystitis or cholangitis, occasionally in association with cryptosporidiosis.

In a similar way to the gastrointestinal tract, CMV infection of the respiratory tract may occur alone or more commonly concurrent with other opportunist pathogens such as *Pneumocystis carinii* or mycobacteria (Murray *et al.*, 1984). This has made some investigators question the role of CMV in pneumonitis in AIDS. There are no particular features of CMV infection of the respiratory tract. However, CMV pneumonitis is usually interstitial rather than alveolar with a diffuse distribution although sometimes apparently focal or lobar involvement occurs. Cultures of CMV from bronchial washings can be difficult to interpret as contamination of the bronchoscope by virus shed in the throat is common. The presence of inclusion bodies in cells or growth of CMV from lung biopsy is of greater relevance.

CMV has also been implicated as the cause of the adrenal insufficiency syndrome observed in some AIDS patients, and post-mortem studies have revealed necrosis of the adrenal glands, particularly in the medulla, in association with evidence of CMV infection (Niedt & Schinella, 1985). Whether CMV accounts for the cases of adrenal insufficiency observed is not yet clear (Greene *et al.*, 1984).

In addition to the direct organ damage caused by CMV the immunosuppressive effects of this virus may add to the immune deficiency. In our experience treatment of CMV has occasionally been associated with regression of disease caused by other opportunist infections without specific treatment. This suggests that an improvement in the general immune status is possible after control of CMV infection.

Nature of CMV infection and strain epidemiology

Herpes viruses are known to establish latent or persistent infections in their hosts. In the case of herpes simplex virus (HSV), the sites of latency are the ganglia in particular

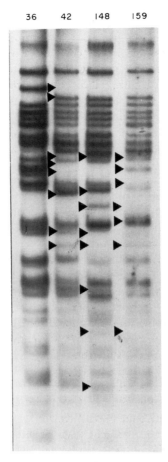

Figure 1. Clinical isolates of CMV were expanded by 4–6 passages in human embryo fibroblasts before infected cells were exposed to ^{32}P-orthophosphate (Amersham). Viral DNA was extracted and analysed by agarose gel electrophoresis after digestion with Sma-1 (Taylor *et al.*, 1988). Restriction profiles for DNA from four clinical isolates (36, 42, 148 and 159), obtained from four different AIDS patients are shown. The marked bands indicate regions of the autoradiograph where differences are evident when the DNA profile is compared to the profile on its left.

those associated with the sensory nerves. Much less is known about CMV although cellular reservoirs appear to exist in salivary glands, prostate and testis and possibly virus is harboured in peripheral blood lymphocytes including macrophages (Jordan, 1983). Reactivation of endogenous CMV is common in immunocompromised individuals but reinfections with exogenous strains of CMV can also occur (Grundy, Super & Griffiths, 1986; Chou, 1986). It might be expected that individuals in a risk group for AIDS would be prone to reinfection with CMV due to (a) repeated exposure to the virus through sexual contact or infected blood and (b) the impending immunodeficiency caused by either HIV or possibly by previous CMV infection. The presence of intermittent IgM antibody to CMV in 95% of IgG-seropositive, male homosexuals over an average period of 14 months was evidence for either frequent reactivation of endogenous virus or constant re-exposure to exogenous virus (Mintz *et al.*, 1983). It has been indicated that multiple strains of CMV can be isolated from

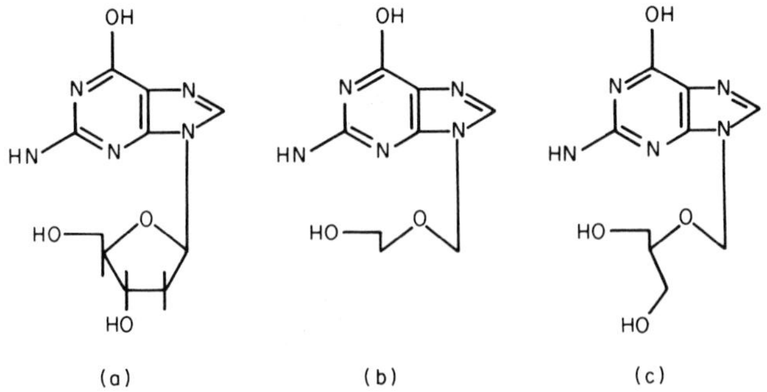

Figure 2. Formulae of acyclic nucleosides (a) 2'-deoxyguanosine, (b) 9(2-hydroxyethoxymethyl) guanine (acyclovir), (c) 9-(1,3-dihydroxy-2-propoxymethyl) guanine (ganciclovir).

patients with AIDS (Drew *et al.*, 1984; Spector, Hirata & Neuman, 1984) but limited information has been published on the strain epidemiology of CMV in this group. We have recently characterized multiple isolates of CMV recovered from AIDS patients by DNA analysis to (a) establish an association of particular strains with the syndrome and (b) to investigate strain heterogeneity within individual patients.

DNA restriction enzyme analysis was used to investigate 37 isolates of CMV obtained from 20 promiscuous homosexual men either suffering from AIDS at the time of virus isolation or who developed AIDS subsequently. Representative viruses from individual patients exhibited major differences in restriction profiles and no one particular strain could be associated with AIDS. These differences are illustrated in Figure 1 which shows DNA restriction profiles for four isolates of CMV obtained from different AIDS patients. Isolates of CMV were obtained from nine patients in the study group either from different sites at the same time or from the same site on different dates. In the case of seven of these men, sequential isolates showed only minor differences in restriction profiles with three or more enzymes and this was interpreted as representing subpopulations of one endogenous strain of CMV. In only two of the nine patients were sufficient differences seen in consecutive isolates to suggest that reinfection with different strains had occurred. It was concluded from this study that although reinfections with CMV in AIDS patients can occur, the isolation of strains exhibiting only minor differences in genome structure was more usual (Taylor *et al.*, 1988).

Antiviral chemotherapy of CMV infection

Ganciclovir

A number of studies on the effectiveness of acyclovir against CMV infections *in vitro* established a range of drug-sensitivities for this compound and analogues about 100-fold lower than established against HSV (Tyms, Scamans & Naim, 1981; Plotkin, Starr & Bryan, 1982). Subsequent clinical trials of acyclovir in patients with CMV disease confirmed the ineffectiveness of acyclovir *in vivo* although results did show some variability (Balfour, 1984). The lack of potency against CMV appears to be a result of limited phosphorylation of the drug and related to the failure of the virus to encode a thymidine kinase activity.

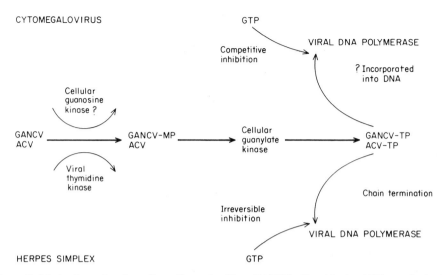

Figure 3. Mechanism of action of acyclic nucleosides. GANCV; Ganciclovir, ACV; acyclovir, GTP; guanosine triphosphate, MP; monophosphate, TP; triphosphate.

Investigation of other compounds with a structure similar to acyclovir (Figure 2) established a broader spectrum of antiviral activity to include potent effect against CMV infections. Ganciclovir, (9(1,3-dihydroxypropoxymethyl) guanine), has in-vitro activity about 50-times greater than acyclovir against CMV and its effectiveness in controlling CMV infections in AIDS patients (see below) has substantiated the predictions made from the in-vitro observations.

We have examined the in-vitro sensitivity to ganciclovir of thirty clinical isolates from nineteen patients attending the STD clinic at St. Mary's Hospital. ED_{50} values for the drug were in the range $0·11–1·10$ μM (D. L. Taylor, unpublished data). ED_{50} values for AD169 ($1·00–1·60$ μM) and Towne ($0·32–1·20$ μM), laboratory strains used as controls, were consistent with those established in a number of studies (Cheng *et al.*, 1983; Tyms *et al.*, 1984; Plotkin *et al.*, 1985). In the course of our work, levels of ganciclovir were verified by spectrophotometric analysis.

Mechanism of antiviral action of ganciclovir

The mechanism of action of ganciclovir with respect to HSV is similar to that described for acyclovir (Figure 3), the increased antiviral effect of ganciclovir correlating with the more efficient formation of di- and triphosphate derivatives by cellular guanylate kinases (Field *et al.*, 1983). The superior antiviral effect of ganciclovir against CMV growth is also related to the increased formation of the monophosphate, almost certainly achieved by cellular enzymes (Biron *et al.*, 1985). Cytosol deoxyguanosine kinase activity from CMV infected cells was inhibited by ganciclovir and the drug was partially phosphorylated by a mitochondrial deoxyguanosine kinase purified from calf thymus (Smee, 1985). In common with HSV, the closer resemblance of ganciclovir to deoxyguanosine appears to favour production of the triphosphate derivative (Field *et al.*, 1983; Smee *et al.*, 1983). CMV-encoded DNA polymerase had greater binding affinity for acyclovir triphosphate (Ki 8 nM) than ganciclovir triphosphate (Ki 22 nM) but both were 7 to 12 times higher than for cellular α-polymerase (Mar *et al.*, 1985).

The lack of cross-resistance of HSV thymidine kinase and DNA polymerase mutants to acyclovir and ganciclovir (Cheng *et al.*, 1983) suggests important differences in the mode of action of acylic nucleosides. The preferential phosphorylation of these compounds is the most critical step in the antiviral action but undoubtedly this is achieved in different ways for different viruses. The cellular phosphorylating activities which appear capable of activating these drugs for action against human CMV and Epstein-Barr virus (Fiddian *et al.*, 1984) replication may also influence the potency against HSV infections. Acyclovir or ganciclovir were between 10- and 100-fold more effective in continuous (Collins & Oliver, 1985) and primary (B. K. Rawal & A. S. Tyms, unpublished results) mouse cells when compared to primate vero cells. This was reflected by the potency of acyclovir against murine CMV *in vitro* (Tyms *et al.*, 1981) and *in vivo* (Burns *et al.*, 1982). Thymidine kinase activity is significantly increased after murine CMV infection of primary mouse cells (Naim & Tyms, 1981) but this activity appeared not to be viral-encoded and probably plays no part in the activation of acyclovir (Burns *et al.*, 1981).

The similarity in structure of ganciclovir to deoxyguanosine particularly the availability of an extra carbon in the sugar moiety analogous to a 3′ deoxyribose appears to enable incorporation of the nucleotide into the growing polynucleotide chain (Frank, Chiou & Cheng, 1984). In contrast, the incorporation of acyclovir monophosphate by viral DNA polymerase caused irreversible inactivation of the enzyme with chain termination (Furman, St. Clair & Spector, 1984). This irreversible-type inhibition by acyclovir triphosphate provides potential advantage but likewise the retention of the phosphorylated derivatives of ganciclovir but not acyclovir in virus infected cells also appears to be a favourable feature (Biron *et al.*, 1985). This effect, which was dose-dependent and most evident at late stages of virus growth, may be a critical factor for enhancing the antiviral response *in vivo*.

Foscarnet (phosphonoformate)

Phosphonoformate (foscarnet), like its analogue phosphonoacetate, has structural similarities to pyrophosphate and competitively inhibits viral DNA polymerase activities of HSV type 1 and type 2 (Cheng *et al.*, 1981) and human CMV (Wahren *et al.*, 1985). Herpes virus encoded DNA polymerases have greater affinity for foscarnet than do cellular α-polymerase but the therapeutic index is narrow (Cheng *et al.*, 1981). The mode of action of this drug may be complex: for example it is known to inhibit also the induction of viral DNA polymerase along with viral DNA-ase activities (Cheng *et al.*, 1981). Foscarnet is a more potent inhibitor of HSV growth than phosphonoacetate and irreversibly inhibits CMV replication *in vitro* (Wahren & Oberg, 1980; Tyms *et al.*, 1987).

Clinical efficacy of antiviral agents in the treatment of CMV disease in patients with AIDS

Several agents have been used in the treatment of CMV disease including ganciclovir, foscarnet, vidarabine, acyclovir and alpha-interferon. Of these only ganciclovir and foscarnet (see below) have demonstrated consistently encouraging results, the

Table II. Efficacy of ganciclovir

Author	No. of patients	Dose (mg/kg)	Frequency/ duration		eye	Response GI tract	lung
1. Collaborative Study Group (1986)	26	5	8–12 hourly 14 days	I I/S	9/13 11/13	5/8	3/7
2. Laskin et al. (1987	97	2·5	8-hourly 14 days	I I/S	30/57 52/57	8/15 9/15	8/20 10/20
3. Jeffries & Pinching (unpublished)	26	2·5–5·0	12-hourly 14 days	I I/S	5/13 12/13	3/4 3/4	4/9 4/9
4. Chachoua et al. (1987)	41	5	12-hourly 14 days	I	—	30/41[a]	—
5. Holland et al. (1986)	20	2·5	8-hourly 10–20 days	I/S	19/20	—	—

[a] 18/41 with complete response of symptoms.
I, Improved; I/S, improved/stabilized.

remainder having little or no effect on CMV disease at tolerable doses (Ch'ien et al., 1974; Balfour et al., 1982; Chou et al., 1984) and will not be further discussed. Hyperimmune anti-CMV immunoglobulin has demonstrated some efficacy in reducing the mortality due to CMV pneumonitis in bone marrow transplant patients but this finding has not been demonstrated in other studies (Reed et al., 1987) and results of its use in AIDS have been disappointing. In contrast, anti-CMV agents such as ganciclovir which have demonstrated some efficacy in pneumonitis in AIDS patients, have not improved the outcome of the same disease in recipients of BMT despite the eradication of active viral replication in the lungs (Shepp et al., 1985; Singer et al., 1985). It is possible that this variation in response is due to different pathogenetic mechanisms operating in these groups of patients. It has been suggested that the pneumonitis in BMT recipients is a result of the immune response to CMV rather than direct damage by the virus (Grundy, Shanley & Griffiths, 1987). This would explain why these patients respond to immunoglobulin which may have some immunomodulating activity. Conversely, patients with AIDS may mount a poor immune response to the virus and disease may therefore be more directly related to viral pathogenicity, with or without other opportunist infection at the site.

Ganciclovir

Ganciclovir is an investigational drug which has been widely used for the treatment of life-threatening or sight-threatening disease due to CMV in patients with AIDS since 1985 (Bach et al., 1985; Collaborative DHPG Study Group, 1986; Felsenstein et al., 1985; Masur et al., 1986). Placebo-controlled trials have not however beeperformed and therefore its efficacy has been judged in comparison with historical controls, and this must be taken into account in its evaluation. However, diseases such as CMV retinitis which respond clinically in >75% patients treated had not previously been found to regress spontaneously and the close correlation between clinical and

Table III. Relapse of CMV disease after stopping ganciclovir

	Incidence	Time to relapse
Collaborative Study Group (1986)		
total	11/14	
retinitis	5/7	2–6 weeks
colitis	4/5	2–14 weeks
pneumonitis	2/3	
Laskin *et al.* (1987)	32/44	
Chachoua *et al.* (1987)	13/33	Median 9 weeks

virological response to ganciclovir (Collaborative DHPG Study Group, 1986) corroborates the clinical impression of its efficacy.

At present the only formulation of ganciclovir routinely used is intravenous (iv). Oral preparations are hampered by poor absorption necessitating large doses. Intravitreal therapy has also been used in a small number of patients in an attempt to overcome the myelotoxicity of systemic therapy. Several centres have reported their results using varying dosage regimens of iv ganciclovir (5·0–15·0 mg/kg per day) (Table II). Studies 1, 2, 4 and 5 were open which makes comparison of response rates difficult. Study 3 is part of a larger double-blind study comparing two dose levels (2·5 and 5·0 mg/kgbd) and these results show a trend to greater response at the higher dose. At 5·0 mg/kg twice daily 16/22 patients responded (73%) compared to 13/21 (62%) (S. A. Danner, D. J. Jeffries & A. J. Pinching, unpublished results). The overall response in different centres has been very similar; combining the results from the studies quoted in Table II, the best outcome has been in the treatment of retinitis and gastro-intestinal tract disease with response (improvement/stabilization) in 94/103 (91%) of retinitis and 46/68 (69%) of intestinal disease. The experience with pneumonitis has been more disappointing with only a 47% response, and many patients dying before completion of the initial course of treatment. There has been very little experience in the treatment of CMV-related nervous system disease, but ganciclovir has not been successful in our experience of encephalitis. Whether this reflects true failure or concurrent HIV encephalopathy is difficult to determine as the two conditions are likely to occur together in many patients.

Virological response tended to precede the clinical response occurring in the study by Laskin *et al.* (1987) at a median of 3·0, 3·5 and 5·0 days in blood, urine and throat cultures respectively. Overall studies showed 70–80% of sites positive on culture for CMV became consistently negative on treatment. The time to clinical response is more variable. Regression of systemic features such as fever, rigor and lymphadenopathy tends to occur early in a similar time period to the virological response and is likely to reflect the loss of viraemia. Evidence of response and healing at disease sites is, as would be expected, more prolonged. In the study by Laskin the median time to stabilization of retinitis was 12·3 days (range 4–31). Holland *et al.* (1986) reported that all patients in their study had stabilized retinitis by day 20 but some patients were noted to have initial deterioration in the first 10 days although this did not appear to compromise their long-term outcome.

Like the other drugs used in the treatment of CMV, ganciclovir does not eradicate

Table IV. Incidence of neutropenia in patients treated with ganciclovir

	Neutrophils $<1\cdot0 \times 10^9/l$	
Jeffries & Pinching (unpublished)	4/26	(15·4%)
Collaborative Study Group (1986)	6/26	(23·0%)
Chachoua *et al.* (1987)	6/26	(23·0%)
Holland *et al.* (1986)	5/20	(25·0%)
Leskin *et al.* (1987)	53/97	(54·6%)

the virus but inhibits replication. Relapse is therefore common (Table III) and will occur in nearly all patients at some time if they do not succumb to another opportunist infection. In our experience it is rare for CMV retinitis or colitis to remain quiescent for longer than 12 weeks and often it will recur much more rapidly. The time to first relapse may depend partly on the decrease in viral load achieved during initial treatment. The double-blind study performed at our centre showed that there was a significant increase in time to recurrence in patients with retinitis treated with 5·0 mg/kg vs 2·5 mg/kg twice daily. Patients on the lower dose relapsed (4/4) within four weeks of completion of the first course of therapy (median three weeks) compared to 1/6 at the high dose (median six weeks) ($P = 0\cdot02$). The high rate of relapse means that maintenance therapy is necessary to prevent recurrent disease. This is particularly the case in retinitis where sight may be lost very rapidly if relapse occurs despite immediate initiation of treatment. Optimal schedules for maintenance ganciclovir have not yet been ascertained and to date comparisons of doses and frequency have only been made on small numbers of patients. However, Laskin (1987) showed that of eight patients with retinitis treated with 5·0 mg/kg 5–7 times per week none relapsed, whereas of those receiving 2·5 mg/kg 3–5 times weekly 11/15 (73%) relapsed and of 21 patients not given maintenance all relapsed. Although it is not clear over what time period these patients were studied or whether the groups were clinically comparable it appears that the higher dosage is superior. It is, important however, to find the minimum dose and frequency of maintenance therapy that gives adequate response rates; ganciclovir is myelosuppressive, and this appears to be cumulative in some patients on long term therapy. Neutropenia will further immunocompromise the patient. In addition to this there are the problems associated with long-term intravenous therapy. Despite the reports of home therapy in many cases this may not be possible, and the necessity of visiting the hospital five days a week for infusion of drug limits the quality of life. Venous access may be a problem and infection of indwelling lines has been troublesome (M. Helbert, personal communication). Owing to the fact that alternative forms of administration are not yet reliable it appears that maintenance with iv ganciclovir will remain the major form of long-term therapy. There is a need to develop regimens that are effective and acceptable to the patient.

Even on full treatment or maintenance ganciclovir some patients will fail to respond, or more commonly relapse (O'Donnell, Jacobson & Mills, 1987). It is possible that this is due to the emergence of resistant virus, however in our experience resistance has not been documented in patients who respond poorly and is more often related to the underlying immune status. It has also been noted in our studies and others (Holland *et al.*, 1986) that in patients with CMV retinitis visual acuity often continues to decline gradually despite apparently inactive disease and maintenance therapy.

In man the most common toxic effect of ganciclovir is on the marrow with 15 to 55% of recipients developing moderate or severe neutropenia ($<1\cdot0$ neutrophils x $10^9/l$) (Table IV). This is reversible but may take one to three weeks to recover on stopping medication. As the effect is dose dependent, cessation of therapy is not always necessary and a temporary decrease in dose may allow the count to recover sufficiently for therapy to continue. It is of interest that the incidence of neutropenia is very different between centres even in those using similar dosage regimens. This may reflect the concurrent use of other drugs, with additional bone marrow toxicity, for treatment or prophylaxis of opportunist infections. Thrombocytopenia and anaemia may also occur but are less common. Of note was the association of increased incidence of severe anaemia in patients on zidovudine and ganciclovir compared to those on zidovudine alone (M. Helbert, D. Robinson, B. Peddle, A. J. Pinching, unpublished results) although this is not generally a reason to discontinue either drug. Other possible side-effects that have been noted with ganciclovir are episodes of confusion, rashes, thrombophlebitis at the site of infusion and nausea.

Inhibition of spermatogenesis observed in animals is worrying but at present there are few data on this possible side-effect in man. Studies on testosterone, follicle-stimulating and luteinizing hormones before and after therapy have not to date shown any consistent change, suggesting that testicular atrophy is not occurring in the short term. However, more detailed investigation of gonadal function in larger numbers of patients is required.

Foscarnet

This compound has been under investigation against herpesvirus infections for some time. Recently, the report of anti-reverse transcriptase activity has encouraged trials of foscarnet as an anti-HIV agent. Although much less has been published on foscarnet for the treatment of CMV in AIDS, recent trials of the drug have been encouraging. The efficacy of foscarnet in one study of CMV retinitis was comparable to that of ganciclovir with five of ten patients showing complete resolution and ten of ten demonstrating improved or stabilized disease (Walmsley *et al.*, 1987). The relapse rate and time to relapse were also comparable with those for ganciclovir and did not confirm earlier suggestions that more prolonged remissions may be achieved (Singer *et al.*, 1985). Foscarnet may also be of value in the treatment of CMV pneumonitis. A small study by Farthing *et al.* (1987a) demonstrated improvement in all eight patients with culture positive CMV pneumonitis within two weeks of starting treatment. However only three patients had complete resolution of symptoms and chest X-ray signs, and all of these had concurrent Pneumocystis carinii infection treatment of which may have led to the observed clinical response. There are anecdotal reports of the response of gastro-intestinal tract disease to this agent (Weber *et al.*, 1986) but our experience suggests it is not as effective as ganciclovir at this site. Major disadvantages of foscarnet are the short half-life and poor CNS penetration necessitating continuous infusion during the course of treatment. If similar administration is necessary for adequate maintenance then this will be a great disadvantage. The need to infuse via a central rather than peripheral vein because thrombophlebitis is also a drawback although the use of diluted infusions may overcome the problem to some extent. In favour of foscarnet is the lack of myelotoxicity which makes it an alternative treatment for patients unable to tolerate ganciclovir. These numbers are likely to become greater with the more widespread use of zidovudine. Side-effects are generally less of a problem with foscarnet compared to ganciclovir although reversible renal impairment with increased serum creatinine levels probably due to toxic tubulopathy has been documented (Ringden *et al.*, 1986). Other reported effects are a decrease in haemoglobin, abnormalities in liver function tests and raised calcium levels (Ringden *et al.*, 1986). The anti-HIV activity of foscarnet may also be of value not only in reducing viral replication and the production of immunosuppressive viral proteins (Farthing *et al.*, 1987*b*) but also theoretically in reducing the effect of HIV in enhancing CMV expression (Skolnik *et al.*, 1988).

Acknowledgements

We are grateful to Dr A. J. Pinching for his helpful comments and wish to thank Syntex Research for support on the clinical and virological studies carried out at St. Mary's Hospital.

References

Apperley, J. F., Marcus, R. E., Goldman, J. M., Wardle, D. G., Gravett, P. J. & Chanas, A. (1985). Foscarnet for cytomegalovirus pneumonitis. *Lancet i*, 1151.

Bach, M. C., Bagwell, S. P., Knapp, N. P., Davis, K. M. & Hedstrom, P. S. (1985). 9-(1,3-dihydroxy-2-propoxymethyl) guanine for cytomegalovirus infections in patients with the acquired immunodeficiency syndrome. *Annals of Internal Medicine* **103**, 381–2.

Bagley, P. H., Scott, D. A., Smith, L. S. & Schillaci, R. F. (1986). Cytomegalovirus infection, ascending myelitis, and pulmonary embolus. *Annals of Internal Medicine,* **104,** 587.

Balfour, H. H. (1984). Acyclovir and other chemotherapy for herpes group viral infections. *Annual Reviews of Medicine* **35,** 279–91.

Balfour, H. H. Jr., Bean, B., Mitchell, C. D., Sachs, G. W., Boen, J. R. & Edelman, C. K. (1982). Acyclovir in immunocompromised patients with cytomegalovirus disease: a controlled trial at one institution. *American Journal of Medicine* **73**, 241–8.

Betts, R. F. (1982). Cytomegalovirus infection in transplant patients. *Progress in Medical Virology* **28,** 44–64.

Biron, K. K., Stanat, S. C., Surrell, J. B., Fyfe, J. A., Keller, P. M., Lambe, C. U. *et al.* (1985). Metabolic activation of the nucleoside analog 9-([2-hydroxy-1-(hydroxymethyl) ethoxy]methy) guanine in human diploid fibroblasts infected with human cytomegalovirus. *Proceedings of the National Academy of Sciences USA* **82**, 2767–70.

Burns, W. H., Wingard, J. R., Bender, W. J. & Sataral, R. (1981). Thymidine kinase not required for antiviral activity of acyclovir against mouse cytomegalovirus. *Journal of Virology* **39**, 889–93.

Burns, W. H., Wingard, J. R., Sandford, G. R., Bender, W. J. & Saral, R. (1982). Acyclovir in mouse cytomegalovirus infections. *American Journal of Medicine* **73** (1A), 118–124.

Carney, W. P., Rubin, R. H., Hoffman, R. A., Hansen, W. P., Healey, K. & Hirsch, M. S. (1981). Analysis of T lymphocyte subsets in cytomegalovirus mononucleosis. *Journal of Immunology* **126**, 2114–6.

Chachoua, A., Dieterich, D., Krasinski, K., Greene, J., Laubenstein, L., Wernz, J. *et al.* (1987). 9-(1,3-dihydroxy-2-proxymethyl) guanine (ganciclovir) in the treatment of cytomegalovirus gastrointestinal disease with the acquired immunodeficiency syndrome. *Annals of Internal Medicine* **107**, 133–7.

Cheng, Y.-C., Grill, S., Derse, D., Chen, J.-Y., Caradonna, S. J. & Conner, K. (1981). Mode of action of phosphonoformate as an anti-herpes simplex virus agent. *Biochemica et Biophysica Acta* **652**, 90–8.

Cheng, Y.-C., Huang, E.-S., Lin, J.-C., Mar, E.-C., Pagano, J. S., Dutschman, G. E. & Grill, S. P. (1983). Unique spectrum of activity of 9-((1,3-dihydroxy-2-propoxy)methyl) guanine against herpesviruses in vitro and its mode of action against herpes simplex virus type 1. *Proceedings of the National Academy of Science USA* **80**, 2767–770.

Chi'en, L. T., Cannon, N. J., Whitley, R. J., *et al.* (1974). Effect of adenine arabinoside on cytomegalovirus infections. *Journal of Infectious Diseases* **130**, 32–9.

Chou, S. (1986). Acquisition of donor strains of cytomegalovirus by renal transplant recipients. *New England Journal of Medicine* **314**, 1418–23.

Chou, S. W., Dylewski, J. S., Gaynon, M. W., Egbert, P. R. & Merigan, T. C. (1984). α-Interferon administration in cytomegalovirus retinitis. *Antimicrobial Agents and Chemotherapy* **25**, 25–8.

Chretien, J. H., McGinniss, C. G. & Muller, A. (1977). Venereal causes of cytomegalovirus mononucleosis. *Journal of the American Medical Association* **238**, 1644–5.

Collaborative DHPG Treatment Study Group (1986). Treatment of serious cytomegalovirus infections with 9-(1,3-dihydroxy-2-propoxymethyl) guanine in patients with AIDS and other immunodeficiencies. *New England Journal of Medicine* **314**, 801–5.

Collins, P. & Oliver, N. M. (1985). Comparison of the in vitro and in vivo antiherpes virus activities of the acyclic nucleosides, acyclovir (zovirax) and 9-((2-hydroxy-1-hydroxy-methylethoxy)methyl) guanine (BWB759U). *Antiviral Research* **5**, 145–56.

Drew, W. L., Mintz, L., Miner, R. C., Sands, M. & Ketterer, B. (1981). Prevalence of cytomegalovirus infection in homosexual men. *Journal of Infectious Diseases* **143**, 188–92.

Drew, W. L., Sweet, E. S., Miner, R. C. & Mocarski, E. S. (1984). Multiple infections by cytomegalovirus in patients with acquired immunodeficiency syndrome: Documentation by southern blot hybridization. *Journal of Infectious Diseases* **150**, 952–3.

Edwards, R. H., Mesing, R. & McKendall, R. R. (1985). Cytomegalovirus meningoencephalitis in a homosexual man with Kaposi's sarcoma: isolation of CMV from CSF cells. *Neurology* **35**, 560–2.

Farthing, C., Anderson, M. G., Ellis, M. E., Gazzard, G. & Chanas, A. C. (1987a). Treatment of cytomegalovirus pneumonitis with foscarnet (trisodium phosphonoformate) in patients with AIDS. *Journal of Medical Virology* **22**, 157–62.

Farthing, C. F., Dalgleish, A. G., Clark, A., McClure, M., Chanas, A. & Gazzard, B. G. (1987b). Phosphonoformate (Foscarnet): a pilot study in AIDS and AIDS related complex. *AIDS* **1**, 21–5.

Felsenstein, D., D'amico, D. J., Hirsch, M. S., Neumeyer, D. A., Cederberg, D. M., De Miranda, P. *et al.* (1985). Treatment of cytomegalovirus retinitis with 9-(2-hydroxy-1-(hydroxymethyl) ethoxymethyl) guanine. *Annals of Internal Medicine* **103**, 377–80.

Fiddian, A. P., Brigden, D., Yeo, J. M. & Hickmott, E. A. (1984). Acyclovir: an update of the clinical applications of this antiherpes agent. *Antiviral Research* **4**, 99–117.

Field, A. K., Davies, M. E., DeWitt, C., Perry, H. C., Liou, R., Germershausen, J. *et al.* (1983). 9-((2-hydroxy-1-(hydroxymethyl)ethoxy)methyl) guanine: A selective inhibitor of herpes group virus replication. *Proceedings of the National Academy of Sciences USA* **80**, 4138–43.

Frank, K. B., Chiou, J.-F. & Cheng, Y.-C. (1984). Interactions of herpes simplex virus-induced DNA polymerase with 9-(1,3-dihydroxy-2-propoxymethyl) guanine triphosphate. *Journal of Biological Chemistry* **259**, 1566–9.

Friedman, A. H., Drellana, J., Freeman, W. R., Luntz, M., Starr, M. B., Tapper, M. L. *et al.* (1983). Cytomegalovirus retinitis: a manifestation of the acquired immune deficiency syndrome (AIDS). *British Journal of Ophthalmology* **67**, 372–80.

Furman, P. A., St Clair, M. H. & Spector, T. (1984). Acyclovir triphosphate is a suicide inactivator of the herpes simplex virus DNA polymerase. *Journal of Biological Chemistry* **259**, 9575–9.

Greenberg, S. B., Linder, S., Baxter, B., Faris, E., Marcus, D. M. & Dreesman, G. (1984). Lymphocyte subsets and urinary excretion of cytomegalovirus among homosexual men attending a clinic for sexually transmitted diseases. *Journal of Infectious Diseases* **150**, 330–3.

Greene, L. W., Cole, W., Greene, J. B., Levy, B., Louie, E., Raphael, B. *et al.* (1984). Adrenal insufficiency as a complication of the acquired immunodeficiency syndrome. *Annals of Internal Medicine* **101,** 497–8.

Griffiths, P. D., Panjwani, D. D., Strik, P. R., Ball, M. G., Ganczakowski, M., Blacklock, H. A. et al. (1984). Rapid diagnosis of cytomegalovirus infection in immunocompromised patients by detection of early antigen fluorescent foci. *Lancet ii,* 1242–5.

Grundy, J. E., Shanley, J. D. & Griffiths, P. D. (1987). Is cytomegalovirus interstitial pneumonitis in transplant recipients an immunopathological condition? *Lancet ii,* 996–9.

Grundy, J. E., Super, M. & Griffiths, P. D. (1986). Reinfection of a seropositive allograft recipient by cytomegalovirus from donor kidney. *Lancet i,* 159–60.

Handsfield, H. H., Chandler, S. H., Caine, V. A., Meyers, J. D., Corey, L., Medeiros, E. et al. (1985). Cytomegalovirus infection in sex partners: evidence for sexual transmission. *Journal of Infectious Diseases* **151,** 344–8.

Holland, G. N., Sakamoto, M. J., Hardy, D., Sidikaro, Y., Kreiger, A. E., Frenkei, L. M. et al. (1986). Treatment of cytomegalovirus retinopathy in patients with acquired immunodeficiency syndrome. *Archives of Ophthalmology* **104,** 1794–800.

Humphrey, R. C., Parkin, J. M. & Marsh, R. J. (1986). The ophthalmological features of AIDS and AIDS related disorders. *Transactions of the Ophthalmological Society of the UK* **105,** 505–9.

Jeantils, V., Lemaitre, M.-O., Robert, J., Gaudouen, Y., Krivitzky, A. & Delzant, G. (1986). Subacute polyneuropathy with encephalopathy in AIDS with human cytomegalovirus pathogenicity? *Lancet ii,* 1039.

Jordan, M. C. (1983). Latent infection and the elusive cytomegalovirus. *Reviews of Infectious Diseases* **5,** 205–15.

Jordan, M. C., Rousseau, W. E., Noble, G. R., Stewart, J. A. & Chin, T. D. Y. (1973). Association of cervical cytomegaloviruses with venereal disease. *New England Journal of Medicine* **288,** 932–4.

Kennedy, P. G. E., Newsome, D. A., Hess, J., Narayan, O. & Suresch, D. L. et al. (1986). Cytomegalovirus but not human T lymphotrophic virus type III/lymphadenopathy associated virus detection by *in situ* hybridisation in retinal lesions in patients with the acquired immune deficiency syndrome. *British Medical Journal* **293,** 162–4.

Lang, D. J. & Kummer, J. F. (1972). Demonstration of cytomegalovirus in semen. *New England Journal of Medicine* **287,** 756–8.

Lang, D. J. & Kummer, J. F. (1975). Cytomegalovirus in semen: observations in selected populations. *Journal of Infectious Diseases* **132,** 472–3.

Laskin, O. L., Cederberg, D. M., Mills, J., Eron, L. J., Mildvan, D. & Spector, S. A. (1987). Ganciclovir for the treatment and suppression of serious infections caused by cytomegalovirus. *American Journal of Medicine* **83,** 201–7.

Leport, C., Harzic, M., Pignon, J. M., Salmon, D., Perrone, C., Bricaire, F. et al. (1987). Benign cytomegalovirus mononucleosis in non-AIDS HIV infected patients. *Lancet ii,* 214.

Mar, E.-C., Chiou, J.-F., Cheng, Y.-C. & Huang, E.-S. (1985). Inhibition of cellular DNA polymerase and human cytomegalovirus-induced DNA polymerase by the triphosphates of 9-(2-hydroxyethoxymethyl) guanine and 9-(1,3-dihydroxy-2-propoxymethyl) guanine. *Journal of Virology* **53,** 776–80.

Masur, H., Lane, C., Palestine, A., Smith, P. D., Manischewitz, J., Stevens, G. et al. (1986). Effect of 9-(1,3-dihydroxy-2-propoxymethyl) guanine on serious cytomegalovirus disease in eight immunosuppressed homosexual men. *Annals of Internal Medicine* **104,** 41–4.

Mintz, L., Drew, W. L., Miner, R. C. & Braff, E. H. (1983). Cytomegalovirus infections in homosexual men. An epidemiological study. *Annals of Internal Medicine* **99,** 326–9.

Moskowitz, L., Hensley, G. T., Chan, J. C. & Adams, K. (1985). Immediate causes of death in acquired immunodeficiency syndrome. *Archives of Pathological Laboratory Medicine* **109,** 735–8.

Murray, J. F., Felton, C. P., Garay, S. M., Gottlieb, M. S., Hopewell, P. C., Stover, D. E. et al. (1984). Pulmonary complications of the acquired immunodeficiency syndrome. *New England Journal of Medicine* **310,** 1682–8.

Myers, J. D., Fleurnoy, N. & Thomas, E. D. (1982). Nonbacterial pneumonia after allogeneic marrow transplantation: a review of ten years' experience. *Reviews of Infectious Diseases* **4,** 1119–32.

Naim, H. M. & Tyms, A. S. (1981). Thymidine kinase activity in mouse embryo fibroblast cells infected with murine cytomegalovirus. *Biochemical and Biophysical Research Communications* **99**, 855–63.

Niedt, G. W. & Schinella, R. A. (1985). Acquired immunodeficiency syndrome. Clinicopathologic study of 56 autopsies. *Archives of Pathological Medicine* **109**, 727–34.

O'Donnell, J. J., Jacobson, M. A. & Mills, J. (1987). Development of cytomegalovirus (CMV) retinitis in a patient with AIDS during ganciclovir therapy for CMV colitis. *New England Journal of Medicine* **316**, 1607–8.

Parkin, J. M., Forster, S. M., Thomson, M., Pinching, A. J. & Jeffries, D. J. (1986). AIDS, cotton wool spots and cytomegalovirus retinitis. *British Medical Journal* **293**, 561–2.

Peckham, C. S., Chin, K. S., Coleman, J. C., Henderson, K., Hurley, R. & Preece, P. M. (1983). Cytomegalovirus infection in pregnancy: preliminary findings from a prospective study. *Lancet i*, 1352–5.

Peterson, P. & Stahl-Bayliss, C. M. (1987). Cytomegalovirus thrombophlebitis after successful DHPG therapy. *Annals of Internal Medicine* **106**, 632–3.

Plotkin, S. A., Drew, W. L., Felsenstein, D. & Hirsch, M. S. (1985). Sensitivity of clinical isolates of human cytomegalovirus to 9-(1,3-dihydroxy-2-propoxymethyl) guanine. *Journal of Infectious Diseases* **152**, 833–4.

Plotkin, S. A., Starr, S. E. & Bryan, C. K. (1982). *In vitro* and *in vivo* responses of cytomegaloviruses to acyclovir. Acyclovir Symposium. *American Journal of Medicine* **731A**, 257–61.

Post, M. J. D., Hensley, G. T., Moskowitz, L. B. & Fischi, M. (1986). Cytomegalic inclusion virus encephalitis in patients with AIDS: CT, clinical and pathologic correlation. *American Journal of Roenterology* **146**, 1229.

Quinn, T. C. (1987). Gastrointestinal manifestations of human immunodeficiency virus. In *Current Topics in AIDS*, Vol. 1 (Gottleib, M. S., Jeffries, D. J., Mildvan, D., Pinching, A. J., Quinn, T. C. & Weiss, R. A., Eds), pp. 155–83. John Wiley.

Reed, E. C., Bowden, R. A., Dandliker, P. S., Gleaves, C. A. & Meyers, J. D. (1987). Efficacy of cytomegalovirus immunoglobulin in marrow transplant recipients with cytomegalovirus pneumonia. *Journal of Infectious Diseases* **156**, 641–4.

Rinaldo, C. R., Carney, W. P., Richter, B. S., Black, P. H. & Hirsch, M. S. (1980). Mechanisms of immunosuppression in cytomegaloviral mononucleosis. *Journal of Infectious Diseases* **141**, 488–95.

Ringden, O., Wilczek, H., Lonnqvist, B., Gahrton, G., Wahren, B. & Lernestedt, J. O. (1985). Foscarnet for cytomegalovirus infections. *Lancet i*, 1503–4.

Ringden, O., Lonnqvist, B., Paulin, T., Ahlmen, V., Klintmalm, G., Wahren, B., *et al.* (1986). Pharmokinetics, safety and preliminary clinical experiences using foscarnet in the treatment of cytomegalovirus infections in bone marrow and renal transplant recipients. *Journal of Antimicrobial Chemotherapy* **17**, 373–87.

Saraux, J. L., Lenoble, L., Toublanc, M. Smiejan, J. M. & Dombret, M. C. (1987). Acalculous cholecystitis and cytomegalovirus infection in a patient with AIDS. *Journal of Infectious Diseases* **155**, 829.

Shepp, D. H., Dandliker, P. S., de Miranda, P., Burnette, T. C., Cederberg, D. M., Kirk, L. E. & Meyers, J. D. (1985). Activity of 9-[2-hydroxy-1-(hydroxymethyl) ethoxymethyl] guanine in the treatment of cytomegalovirus pneumonia. *Annals of Internal Medicine* **103**, 368–73.

Singer, D. R. J., Fallon, T. J., Schulenburg, W. E., Williams, G. & Cohen, J. (1985). Foscarnet for cytomegalovirus retinitis. *Annals of Internal Medicine* **103**,

Skolnik, P. R., Osloff, B. R. & Hirsch, M. (1988). Bidirectional interactions between human immunodeficiency virus type 1 and cytomegalovirus. *Journal of Infectious Diseases* **137**, 508–14.

Smee, D. F. (1985). Interaction of 9-(1,3-dihydroxy-2-propoxymethyl) guanine with cytosol and mitochondrial deoxyguanosine kinases: possible role in anti-cytomegalovirus activity. *Molecular and Cellular Biochemistry* **69**, 75–81.

Smee, D. F., Martin, J. C., Verheyden, J. P. H. & Matthews, T. R. (1983). Anti-herpesvirus activity of the acyclic nucleoside 9-(1,3-dihydroxy-2-propoxymethyl) guanine. *Antimicrobial Agents and Chemotherapy* **23**, 676–82.

Smith, P. D., Lane, H. C., Gill, V. J., Manischewitz, J. F., Quinnan, G. V., Fauci, A. S. & Masur, H. (1988). Intestinal infections in patients with the acquired immunodeficiency syndrome. *Annals of Internal Medicine* **108**, 328–33.

Spector, S. A., Hirata, K. K. & Neuman, T. R. (1984). Identification of multiple cytomegalovirus strains in homosexual men with the acquired immunodeficiency syndrome. *Journal of Infectious Diseases* **150,** 953–5.

Stagno, S., Pass, R. F., Dworsky, M. E. & Alford, C. A. (1982). Maternal cytomegalovirus infection and perinatal transmission. *Clinical Obstetrics and Gynaecology* **25,** 563–77.

Taylor, D. L., Taylor-Robinson, D., Jeffries, D. J. & Tyms, A. S. (1988). Characterisation of cytomegalovirus isolates from patients with AIDS by DNA restriction analysis. *Epidermiology and Infection,* in press.

Tyms, A. S., Davis, J. M., Clarke, J. R. & Jeffries, D. J. (1987). Synthesis of cytomegalovirus DNA is an antiviral target late in virus growth. *Journal of General Virology* **68,** 1563–73.

Tyms, A. S., Davis, J. M., Jeffries, D. J. & Meyers, J. D. (1984). BWB759U, An analogue of acyclovir, inhibits human cyromegalovirus in vitro. *Lancet ii,* 924–5.

Tyms, A. S., Scamans, E. M. & Naim, H. M. (1981). The *in vitro* activity of acyclovir and related compounds against cytomegalovirus infections. *Journal of Antimicrobial Chemotherapy* **8,** 65–72.

Wahren, B., Ruden, U., Gadler, H., Oberg, B. & Eriksson, B. (1985). Activity of the cytomegalovirus genome in the presence of PPi analogs. *Journal of Virology* **56,** 996–1001.

Wahren, B. & Oberg, B. (1980). Reversible inhibition of cytomegalovirus replication by phosphonoformate. *Intervirology* **14,** 7–15.

Walmsley, S. L., Chew, E., Fanning, M. M., Read, S. E., Vellend, H. & Salit, I. E. (1987). Treatment of cytomegalovirus retinitis with phosphonoformate (Foscarnet). Abstract TH8.1., p. 158 *Third International AIDS conference, Washington.*

Weber, J. N., Thom, S., Barrison, I., Unwin, R., Forster, S., Jeffries, D. J., *et al.* (1986). Cytomegalovirus colitis and oesophageal ulceration in the context of AIDS: clinical manifestations and preliminary report of treatment with foscarnet (phosphonoformate). *Gut* **28,** 482–7.

Journal of Antimicrobial Chemotherapy (1989) **23**, *Suppl. A*, 107–125

Fungal and mycobacterial infections in patients infected with the human immunodeficiency virus

Patricia M. Spencer[a] and George Gee Jackson[a,b]

[a]*Department of Medicine, University of Illinois Chicago, Illinois, USA; and*
[b]*Department of Medical Microbiology, The London Hospital Medical College, London, UK*

Fungal and mycobacterial infections are among the most common opportunistic infections in patients infected with human immunodeficiency virus (HIV). Candida infections are the bell-wether of progression to symptomatic HIV infection and candida oesophagitis often marks the onset of the acquired immunodeficiency syndrome (AIDS). More than 80% of AIDS patients have candida disease. Candida infections remain local and respond to treatment but tend to recur. Cryptococcal infections initially affect few HIV positive patients but involve 10–30% with AIDS. Meningitis is the usual presentation and dissemination is common. Amphotericin usually produces improvement but cure is infrequent, and maintenance therapy is advisable. Mycobacteria cause intracellular infections increasing in parallel with immunodeficiency. *Mycobacterium avium-intracellulare* is predominant, occuring with other opportunistic pathogens causing systemic and local symptoms with high bacterial density in infected cells. Multidrug treatment is best, but the results are disappointing. Tuberculosis is prevalent in certain groups of patients. It often presents with atypical clinical and pathological features. Anti-tuberculous treatment is effective and prophylaxis should be considered. Endemic fungi with mycobacteria cause sporadic infections. Opportunistic infections are the lethal arm of HIV infection. Diligent diagnosis and persistent treatment offer benefit to HIV-infected patients.

Introduction

Fungal and mycobacterial infections are among the most common opportunistic infections occurring in adult patients infected with the human immunodeficiency virus (HIV). They are the initial presenting complaint in 3–30% of patients and affect most patients in the course of the acquired immunodeficiency syndrome (AIDS). The infections range in severity from trivial to the precipitating cause of death. The aetiology and sites of infection are influenced by the environmental geography, previous and concomitant infections, and most by the degree of impairment of the immunological systems. The source of the microorganisms is from exogenous exposure or reactivation of intrinsic latent infection. The former is believed to be the mode for fungal infections and the latter for *Mycobacterium tuberculosis*, but either source can apply to either type of infection. Ubiquitous yeasts or endemically prevalent fungi are the predominant causes of fungal infection. The same is true for non-tuberculous mycobacteria; tuberculosis is usually a recrudescent infection. The pathogenesis of disease with fungi and mycobacteria is different; the former are extracellular whilst mycobacteria are intracellular pathogens. The histological features reveal impairment

107

0305–7453/89/23A107 + 19 $02.00/0

of cellular immunity. Local overgrowth or in-situ replication of the infecting species is poorly controlled; immunopathological reactions such as granulomas and caseation are often missing. Abscesses, fungal masses and displacement of normal tissue are local changes, and dissemination is far more common than can be attributed to the primary invasiveness of the organisms or than is found in the same infections when they occur in patients without overt immunodeficiency. These features all affect the clinical syndromes which have a remarkable range of variation with each type of infection.

Candida

Clinical syndromes

Candida species, usually *Can. albicans* are the most common cause of opportunistic infections of patients with AIDS or the AIDS-related complex (ARC), occurring in 80–90% (Holmberg & Meyer, 1986). The clinical categorization of candida infections in HIV infected individuals is shown in Table I. Mucocutaneous candidiasis, which is the most frequent syndrome, is a focal disease. Invasive or disseminated disease which threatens life, is infrequent (Holmberg & Meyer, 1986; Heinemann, Bloom & Horowitz, 1987).

   Mucocutaneous candidiasis. The oropharynx, oesophagus, and vagina are the usual sites of mucocutaneous candida infection. Oral candidiasis alone occurs at some time in 80% of AIDS patients (Welch *et al.*, 1984). It may be an initial sign or a new prognostic feature in previously asymptomatic or ARC patients; 59% of the latter with oral thrush were observed to develop full blown AIDS (Klein *et al.*, 1984). Similarly, a high percentage (24%) of HIV-infected women were found to have chronic refractory vaginal candidiasis; 89% of these women developed AIDS within 30 months of follow-up (Rhoads *et al.*, 1987). Oral and vaginal candida infections appear to occur at the beginning of advancing immunodeficiency. Chronic mucocutaneous candidiasis is known to be associated with defects in cellular immunity against candida. This subtle test of immunological function may explain the high frequency of mucocutaneous candidiasis as the initial manifestation of AIDS (Holmberg & Meyer, 1986; Heinemann *et al.*, 1987). The local infections respond well to therapy, but relapse and reinfection occur frequently after treatment is stopped.

Table I. Candida infections in AIDS

Syndromes	Diagnosis	Treatment	Outcome
I Mucocutaneous (common)	⎰ Typical appearance	Local nystatin or clotrimazole	Treatment successful
Oropharyngeal Vaginal	⎱ KOH preparation Gram stain	Ketoconazole (oral) for refractory cases	Relapse expected
Oesophageal	Endoscopy Candida in brushings or biopsy	Amphotericin B if debilitating; 5-fluorocytosine if tolerated	Symptoms improve. Endoscopic change less likely
II Parenchymal or disseminated (uncommon)	Histology or culture of affected site	Amphotericin B; 5-fluorocytosine and optimal dosage & duration unknown	Data inadequate— some successes

Oesophageal candidiasis. Oesophageal candidiasis was diagnosed in 14% of AIDS patients in the USA (Centers for Disease Control Report, 1986). In contrast to oral and vaginal candidiasis, oesophageal infection is used as a diagnostic sign of AIDS Centers for Disease Control Report, (1987*a*). Systemic dissemination rarely occurs from an oesophageal source (Holmberg & Meyer, 1986). When it is symptomatic, oesophageal candidiasis presents as odynophagia and dysphagia; nausea, vomiting, early satiety and haematemesis are other symptoms (Tavitian, Raufman & Rosenthal, 1986*a, b*; Levine *et al.*, 1987). Some patients with oesophageal candida infection are asymptomatic (Clotet *et al.*, 1986; Tavitian *et al.*, 1986*a*). Oesophageal candidiasis is often the cause in patients who present with oral lesions and dysphagia/odynophagia, although other oesophageal infections are sometimes found in this setting (Tavitian *et al.*, 1986*b*; Levine *et al.*, 1987).

Disseminated candidiasis. In contrast to mucocutaneous candidiasis, invasive candidiasis is infrequently encountered in ARC and AIDS. When it occurs, disseminated candidiasis correlates with neutropenia and neutrophil dysfunction rather than with defects in cell-mediated immunity (Holmberg & Meyer, 1986; Whimbey *et al.*, 1986). Although candida is not a common pulmonary pathogen, the lungs are the most common parenchymal site of infection (Stover *et al.*, 1985; Holmberg & Meyer, 1986). The occurrence of pulmonary candida infection in an HIV-infected patient is another diagnostic criterion for AIDS (Centers for Disease Control Report, 1987*a*). Other tissue infections in disseminated candidiasis include meningitis, brain abscess, endophthalmitis and chorioretinitis, usually associated with disseminated disease (Levy, Bredesen & Rosenblum, 1985; Ehni & Ellison, 1987; Heineman *et al.*, 1987).

Analysis of positive blood cultures in AIDS patients shows that candidaemia does not occur in greater frequency than it does in non-AIDS patients, and the isolation of candida from the blood is usually associated with the presence of an iv catheter (Eng *et al.*, 1986*b*; Whimbey *et al.*, 1986). Disseminated candidiasis is infrequently discovered at autopsy (Reichert *et al.*, 1983; Welch *et al.*, 1984). Cases of disseminated infection found at autopsy in AIDS patients indicate that candida may be hospital acquired, related to the use of broad spectrum antibiotics and indwelling intravenous catheters rather than occurring because of the inherent immune dysfunction (Gold, 1985; Heinemann *et al.*, 1987).

Diagnosis

Mucocutaneous candida infection is diagnosed by observation of a typical lesion, and the demonstration of organisms in a smear or biopsy of the affected tissue. Oral and vaginal candidiasis can be diagnosed by typical clinical presentations (whitish plaques on the oral mucosa or tongue; thick, curd-like vaginal discharge), and confirmed by KOH or Gram stained smears showing candida. A positive culture for candida is not definitive as the oral pharynx may be colonized without this having aetiological importance (Holmberg & Meyer, 1986).

The diagnosis of oesophageal candidiasis is made by endoscopic observation of characteristic whitish plaques, or in some cases, ulcers involving the oesophageal mucosa. Cytological examination of brushings or biopsy material usually reveals an abundance of candida (Figure 1). Oesophageal biopsy can be less sensitive for detecting candida than brushings of the affected areas, owing to the patchy involvement of the tissue.

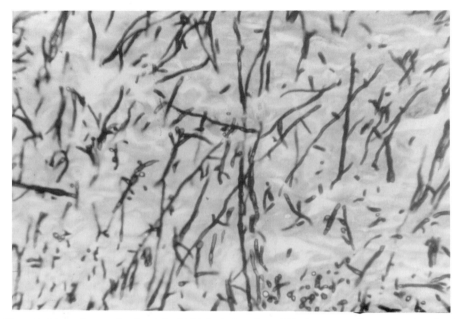

Figure 1. Photomicrograph of a stained histological section of the lower oesophagus showing abundant mycelia and yeast forms of *Can. albicans* in a patient with AIDS and oesophageal candidiasis.

Pulmonary candidiasis must be confirmed by the finding of bronchial plaques and detecting organisms in a stained smear or by histological signs of invasive disease. As in oral candidiasis, positive cultures of the respiratory secretions alone are insufficient basis for the diagnosis of pulmonary candidiasis. The diagnosis of disseminated candidiasis in other organs require histological or cultural evidence of candida in a normally sterile tissue site.

Therapy and outcome

Initial treatment of oral and vaginal candidiasis by local medication, either nystatin, 4–6 million units/day or clotrimazole troches, 10 mg five times/day is frequently successful. For refractory cases, systemic ketoconazole has been used. Response to therapy is usually good, but relapses frequently require retreatment or maintenance therapy in the majority of patients (Holmberg & Meyer, 1986).

The treatment of oesophageal candida is similar to that at other mucosal sites. Oral ketoconazole gives clinical improvement within five days in most patients with oesophageal candidiasis (Tavitian *et al.*, 1986*b*). Endoscopic follow-up of six patients on therapy revealed persistent candida in all patients examined despite clinical improvement. In view of the toxicity of amphotericin, flucytosine and high dose ketoconazole, the risk/benefit and cost/benefit ratios of aggressive therapy for candida oesophagitis are of uncertain value. Patients with extensive oesophageal involvement or those debilitated by the persistent symptoms can be treated with amphotericin B: 10–20 mg/day for 7–10 days has been suggested as adequate therapy (Holmberg & Meyer, 1986). Some patients with very extensive oesophagitis may require amphotericin in higher doses for longer periods of time (Tavitian *et al.*, 1986*b*). The addition of flucytosine has been beneficial in some cases (Farman *et al.*, 1986). Long term maintenance or retreatment is usually required. Control of symptoms rather than

Table II. Characteristic cryptococcal diseases complicating AIDS (University of Illinois, Chicago)

Patient	Clinical syndrome	Diagnostic data			Treatment	Other chronic medications	Outcome
		Cerebrospinal fluid	Other				
30 year-old Hispanic male (HIV positive)	Meningitis without dissemination	5 RBC, 1 WBC/mm^3 Glucose 49 g/dl Protein 56 mg/dl Cryptococcal antigen 1 : 64 Culture positive	Serum antigen 1 : 256 Blood culture negative		Amphotericin B 10 weeks 1200 mg dose	Zidovudine	Cured
32 year-old Black male Homosexual	Meningitis intractable disseminated	10 RBC, 6 WBC/mm^3 Glucose 26 mg/dl Protein 180 mg/dl Cryptococcal antigen 1 : 4096 India ink & culture positive	Serum antigen 1 : 4096 Blood cultures positive		Amphotericin B 5 months > 5000 mg + 5 fluorocytosine	Clotrimazole troche	Died from PCP Persistent cryptococcosis
42 year old Hispanic female Husband, bisexual	Fungaemia, late meningitis	12 RBC, 7 WBC/mm^3 Glucose 44 mg/dl Protein 37 g/dl Cryptococcal antigen 1 : 128 India ink & culture positive	Serum antigen 1 : 256 Blood culture positive		Amphotericin B 6 weeks 1000 mg total	Pyrimethamine Sulphadiazine	Clinically cured Died of other infections
28 year-old White male Homosexual	Pulmonary cryptococcus	No cells Normal fluid Antigen negative Culture negative	Biopsy positive Serum antigen negative Culture negative		Amphotericin B 500 mg Ketoconazole	Zidovudine	Clinically cured

cure is the goal in the treatment of oesophageal candidiasis in AIDS. Individualization of dose and duration of antifungal therapy can be based on the clinical response.

Information about therapy of disseminated candidiasis in AIDS patients is limited and inadequate to define optimal therapy or the expected course following treatment. The combination of amphotericin B and flucytosine has consensus acceptance as the therapy of choice for life threatening invasive candidiasis in patients without AIDS, and on that basis it is recommended. The regimen has been temporarily successful in the treatment of disseminated candidiasis in patients with AIDS (Levy *et al.*, 1985; Ehni & Ellison, 1987).

Cryptococcus

Clinical syndromes

Cryptococcal infections are life-threatening opportunistic infections causing morbidity and mortality in AIDS and other patients with defects in cellular immunity. It is the initial presentation in 3%, and the most common disseminated fungal infection of patients with AIDS (Holmberg & Meyer, 1986). Between 2 and 9% of patients with AIDS in the USA and 29% of those in Africa have cryptococcal infections. Four patients summarized in Table II are illustrative of the spectrum of the clinical syndromes produced by cryptococcal infection in patients with AIDS. All of the patients had had episodes of *Pneumocystis carinii* pneumonia (PCP), and usually candida and herpesvirus infections; diseases such as diabetes were other factors. The multitude of host diseases in patients infected with cryptococcus emphasizes the severity of the immune deficiency and the complex nature of the opportunistic infections.

Meningitis with or without systemic involvement is the most common initial manifestation of cryptococcal infections. In two reported series of documented cryptococcal infections in patients with AIDS, meningitis was the site of infection in 22 of 26, and 18 of 27 (Kovacs *et al.*, 1985; Zuger *et al.*, 1986). Extraneural involvement occurred in about one-half of them. The most frequent sites of dissemination have been lungs, blood, lymph nodes, liver, spleen, kidney, bone marrow and skin, but virtually any organ may be involved (Kovacs *et al.*, 1985; Eng *et al.*, 1986a; Dismukes, 1988). Figure 2 shows a lymph node with extensive tissue replacement by cryptococci. More unusual sites of disseminated cryptococcal disease are the prostate, joints, pericardium, myocardium, peritoneum, adrenals, and thyroid (Kovacs *et al.*, 1985; Lief & Sarfarazi, 1986; Ricciardi *et al.*, 1986; Brivet *et al.*, 1987; LaFont *et al.*, 1987; Witt *et al.*, 1987).

The presentation of cryptococcal disease may be acute or chronic, with the onset of symptoms from one day to four months before diagnosis (Zuger *et al.*, 1986). Headache and fever are signs of the infection in 80–90% of patients with cryptococcal meningitis; photophobia is present in 20–30%, stiff neck in 30%, mental status changes in 20%, and malaise, nausea and vomiting in 40–50% (Kovacs *et al.*, 1985; Zuger *et al.*, 1986). Computer tomography scans of the head of 13 patients with cryptococcal meningitis revealed a cryptococcoma in two, and a hyperdense lesion that resolved with antifungal treatment in a third patient (Zuger *et al.*, 1986).

The lungs are the most common site of non-CNS cryptococcal disease (Dismukes, 1988). A cryptococcoma of the lung, shown as the fourth exemplary syndrome in Table II, has not been previously reported. Other forms of localized disease without

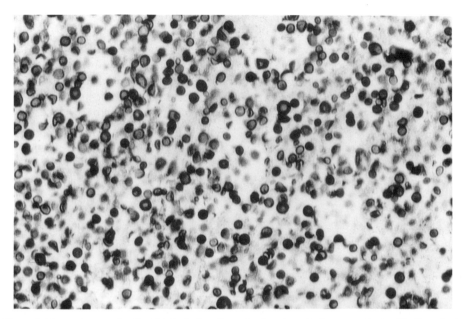

Figure 2. Photomicrograph of a histological section of a lymph node from a patient with disseminated cryptococcosis. Note the marked replacement of lymphocytes and normal lymph node structures by cryptococci.

CNS involvement have been observed (Kovacs *et al.*, 1985; LaFont *et al.*, 1987). The presenting symptoms and signs reflect the specific organ system involved. Cryptococcal infection without symptoms of meningitis or localized disease comprise a distinct subgroup of about 9% of patients with AIDS and cryptococcal infection (Kovacs *et al.*, 1985; Roux *et al.*, 1986; Zuger *et al.*, 1986). These patients may be asymptomatic or have nonspecific complaints, predominantly malaise and fever.

Diagnosis

Examination of the cerebrospinal fluid is necessary to make the diagnosis of cryptococcal meningitis. As shown by the data in Table II patients with AIDS and cryptococcal meningitis usually have normal glucose concentration, slight if any elevation of protein, and few cells in the cerebrospinal fluid (CSF). Cryptococci in the meninges with little cellular reaction are shown in Figure 3. Cryptococcal-specific studies, including antigen detection, staining by India-ink contrast, and isolation of organisms in culture are positive in nearly all of the patients. Cryptococcal antigen is also present in the serum, sometimes with extraordinary high titres of up to 1 : 2,000,000 (Eng *et al.*, 1986). Its presence in the serum has been proposed as a screening test for febrile AIDS patients who have no localizing symptoms (Kovacs *et al.*, 1985; Roux *et al.*, 1986). Positive blood cultures are a characteristic of disseminated cryptococcosis and cultures should be obtained in all patients suspected of infection. A lysis-centrifugation system is recommended (Robinson *et al.*, 1987). Other body fluids or biopsy specimens are also useful for culture and histological examinations.

The diagnosis of pulmonary cryptococcosis is made by bronchoscopy with bronchoalveolar lavage (BAL) and transbronchial biopsy. The sensitivity of BAL for

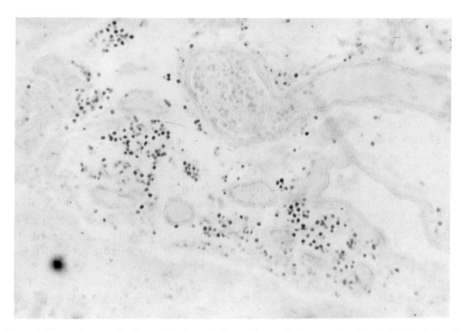

Figure 3. Photomicrograph of a section through the meninges of the second patient in Table II who died with chronic cryptococcal meningitis. Note the cryptococci in the subarachnoid space and minimal cellular infiltration.

Table III. Drugs of choice for deep fungal infections

Infecting organism	Drug of first choice	Alternative drugs
Aspergillus spp.	Amphotericin B with or without flucytosine or rifampicin	No dependable alternative
B. dermatitidis	Ketoconazole or amphotericin B	
Candida spp.	Amphotericin B with or without flucytosine	Ketoconazole
Cocci. immitis	Ketoconazole or amphotericin B	Miconazole
Crypt. neoformans	Amphotericin B with or without flucytosine	No dependable alternative
H. capsulatum	Ketoconazole or amphotericin B	
Mucor spp. and other agents of mucormycosis	Amphotericin B	No dependable alternative
Paracoccidioides brasiliensis	Ketoconazole or amphotericin B	A sulphonamide
Pseudallescheria boydii	Ketoconazole or miconazole	No dependable alternative
Sporothrix schenckii	An iodide	Amphotericin B

From: *The Medical Letter* (1988), **30**, Issue 761.

detecting cryptococcus was 83% by smear and 100% by histological examination of BAL cell blocks in biopsy positive cases (Gal *et al.*, 1986).

Therapy

Drugs considered to be of first choice and alternative treatment for deep fungal infections are given in Table III (The Medical Letter, 1988). As noted in Table II the results of treatment show initial success in the treatment of most patients with cryptococcal infections. But the mortality rate from initial failure is appreciable and ultimate failure from relapses is high. A variety of drugs and dosage regimens have been used. Of 24 patients treated with amphotericin B alone or combined with flucytosine, most patients showed clinical improvement (Kovacs *et al.*, 1985). However, 14 of 24 failed to achieve complete cure and eventually died. Ten patients completed treatment and appeared to be cured but of them six relapsed. Only four patients had sustained clinical improvement after the initial course of therapy, and only one patient improved after a second course. In another series, 18 of 24 patients surviving the first course of therapy were apparently free of disease; relapse occurred in 4 of 8 patients who did not continue with maintenance antifungal therapy (Zuger *et al.*, 1986). All of the patients with relapse died whereas none of seven given 100 mg of amphotericin B weekly as maintenance therapy died of cryptococcal infection.

The results of treatment have not shown a correlation with the initial titre of serum cryptococcal antigen, the demonstration of organisms by India ink or positive cultures. Persistence of cryptococcal antigen in CSF in a titre of 1 : 8 or greater may predict relapse, (Eng *et al.*, 1986*a*; Zuger *et al.*, 1986).

Toxicity to amphotericin B in AIDS patients was not more frequent than expected. Use of flucytosine was restricted in about one-half of patients because of pre-existing leucopenia or impaired renal function. Among those who received flucytosine in addition to amphotericin, the adverse reaction rate was high; one-third required its discontinuation because of haematological abnormalities, abnormal renal or liver function tests or exacerbation of ulcerative colitis.

Considering the poor outcome of cryptococcal infection in patients with AIDS, aggressive antifungal treatment is recommended within the tolerance of the patient. Doses of amphotericin higher than those used in other patients, in the range of 0.5–0.8 mg/kg/day may be advisable. The total dose should be at least 1 g. The role of intrathecal amphotericin B is not clear. Mostly this treatment route has been used in patients failing conventional therapy and the fatality rate is high, although some successes have been reported (Kovacs *et al.*, 1985; Zuger *et al.*, 1986; Dismukes, 1988). If flucytosine is used, monitoring drug levels and haematological indices is essential. Treatment should be continued as long as cultures remain positive. Based on available experience, maintenance doses of amphotericin B once or twice weekly are advisable.

Oral maintenance treatment has been successful in some AIDS patients with cryptococcal meningitis. (Dismukes, 1988). As shown in the chest X-rays before and after treatment, our patient with a pulmonary cryptococcoma responded to oral ketoconazole (Figure 4). Limited penetration of ketoconazole into the CNS decreases its effectiveness in most cryptococcal infections. The Newer triazoles, itraconazole and fluconazole, may have more promise as initial and maintenance therapy of patients with AIDS and cryptococcal infections (Dismukes, 1988).

P. M. Spencer and G. G. Jackson

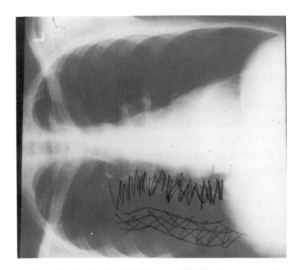

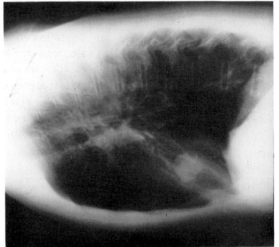

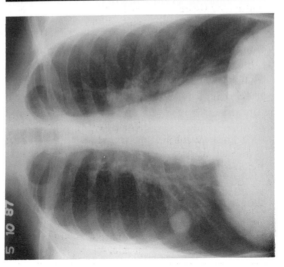

Figure 4. Chest X-ray of a patient with a biopsy proven cryptococcoma in the anterior segment of the right lower lobe of the lung (left and centre). Chest X-ray after brief treatment with amphotericin followed by oral ketoconazole showing disappearance of the fungal mass (right).

Other fungal infections

Virtually all fungi, especially those endemic to particular geographical regions can cause opportunistic infections in patients with AIDS. *Blastomyces, Histoplasma, Coccidioides, Aspergillus* and *Mucor* spp. are among the fungi that have been observed as opportunistic infections in patients with AIDS and must be differentiated from *Candida* and *Cryptococcus* spp. as causes of infection in HIV-infected individuals. Smears, cultures and histological sections usually provide easy differentiation. Aggressive specific treatment and maintenance therapy with the drugs listed in Table III are usually clinically beneficial.

Mycobacterium avium-intracellulare

Clinical syndromes

Myco. avium-intracellulare is ubiquitous in the environment, being found in dust and water. Two major clinical forms of disease are outlined in Table IV. Before the epidemic of AIDS, *Myco. avium-intracellulare* was recognized as a cause of pulmonary infection in older men with chronic lung disease, but disseminated disease was rare (Wollinsky, 1979). The initial reports of disseminated infections due to *Myco. avium-intracellulare* in AIDS were in 1982 (Greene *et al.*, 1982; Zadowski *et al.*, 1982). Since that time, *Myco. avium-intracellulare* infection has become recognized as one of the most common opportunistic infections in patients with AIDS (Macher *et al.*, 1983; Kiehn *et al.*, 1985; Wong *et al.*, 1985; Hawkins *et al.*, 1986). Ante-mortem diagnosis of *Myco. avium-intracellulare* is made in about 20% of AIDS patients but autopsy studies

Table IV. Mycobacterial infections in AIDS

Syndromes	Diagnosis	Treatment	Outcome
Myco. avium-intracellulare			
Disseminated (fever, weight loss, cachexia malaise)	Cultures: blood, bone marrow, stool, sputum, or tissue Histology of infected tissues	Rifabutin plus clofazimine isoniazid ethambutol	Poor Patients die with active disease, (direct contribution to death unclear)
Diarrhoea, malabsorption	Stool AFB smear & culture Sigmoidoscopy, biopsy	Multiple regimens tried	Continues to death
Myco. tuberculosis			
Extrapulmonary (65%)		For all types:	
Nonpulmonary (30%)	AFB smear & culture of infected tissues, secretions or sputum	isoniazid & rifampicin plus	Patients die of other infections
With pulmonary (35%)		pyrazinamide or ethambutol	Generally good response to treatment
Pulmonary (30%)	Chest X-ray (atypical) Bronchoscopy	Continue until cultures negative Six to nine months minimum	

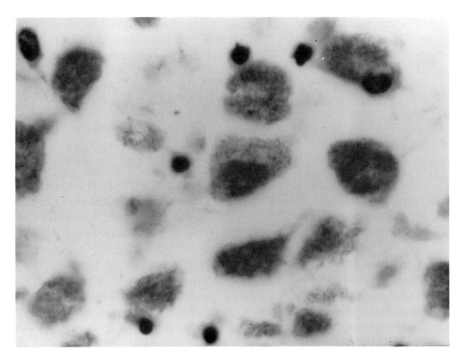

Figure 5. A photomicrograph of cells from the duodenum of a patient with AIDS infected with *Myco. avium-intracellulare.* Note the abundance of organisms (acid fast bacilli) in each infected cell.

indicate that infection may be present in 40–50% of them (Kiehn *et al.,* 1985; Hawkins *et al.,* 1986). Infection with *Myco. avium-intracellulare* often occurs late in the clinical course of AIDS, and is usually accompanied by other opportunistic infections or malignancy.

The clinical symptoms most often ascribed to disseminated *Myco. avium-intracellulare* are vague and non-specific. Fever, anorexia, weight loss and malaise are common, sometimes accompanied by hepatosplenomegaly and lymphadenopathy. The exact role of *Myco. avium-intracellulare* in the symptom complex is not well defined. Organ specific, localized symptoms are the exception (Zakowski *et al.,* 1982; Macher *et al.,* 1983; Kiehn *et al.,* 1985; Wong *et al.,* 1985; Hawkins *et al.,* 1986; Poropatich, Labriola & Tuazon, 1987). Since *Myco. avium-intracellulare* usually accompanies other opportunistic infections such as cytomegalovirus (CMV) infection, or PCP, or a malignancy, it is difficult to ascribe non-specific clinical symptoms only to *Myco. avium-intracellulare.* The large number of acid-fast organisms found in infected tissues lends support to the role of *Myco. avium-intracellulare* in AIDS-associated morbidity (Zakowski *et al.,* 1982; Damsker & Bottone, 1985; Wong *et al.,* 1985; Masur *et al.,* 1987). In disseminated *Myco: avium-intracellulare,* any tissue or organ can be infected: spleen, lymph node, lung, gastrointestinal and genitourinary tracts are the sites often infected (Greene *et al.,* 1982; Zakowski *et al.,* 1982; Hawkins *et al.,* 1986). Many patients are bacteraemic, frequently with continuously positive blood cultures (Macher *et al.,* 1983; Kiehn *et al.,* 1985; Wong *et al.,* 1985).

While non-specific symptoms are the rule in AIDS patients with *Myco. avium-intercellulare,* a subgroup of patients have abdominal pain and diarrhoea as prominent features of infection. The presence of organisms in colonic biopsies correlates with the symptoms (Hawkins *et al.,* 1986). In addition, patients with malabsorption and histological features resembling Whipple's disease have been described (Gillin, Urmacher & West, 1983). The remarkable number of organisms found in tissue in patients with gastrointestinal infection, (Figure 5) has led some investigators to postulate the gut as a source of primary infection (Young *et al.,* 1986; Damsker & Bottone, 1985).

Diagnosis

Myco. avium-intercellulare has been cultured from multiple body fluids and tissues from patients with AIDS. The high frequency of bacteraemia makes blood cultures a particularly useful means of diagnosis; up to 96% of AIDS patients with *Myco. avium-intercellulare* infection have positive blood cultures (Zakowski *et al.,* 1982; Wong *et al.,* 1985; Kiehn *et al.,* 1986). Mycobacterial blood cultures using the lysis centrifugation system can be used to quantitate bacteraemia, and perhaps used to follow the response of patients to therapy (Kiehn *et al.,* 1985; Wong *et al.,* 1985; Young *et al.,* 1986). Positive cultures from respiratory secretions, stool and bone marrow may precede bacteraemia (Hawkins *et al.,* 1986; Poropatich *et al.,* 1987). Urine culture is positive in fewer patients, but liver and lymph node cultures yield a high rate of positive cultures in infected patients (Hawkins *et al.,* 1986; Young *et al.,* 1986). Cultures are often positive when the smear of the specimen is negative (Kiehn *et al.,* 1986).

The diagnosis of *Myco. avium-intracellulare* is made more frequently at autopsy than in life. The indolent nature of the disease, non-specificity of the symptoms and concomitant infections are contributory factors. Suspicion of infection with *Myco. avium-intracellulare* should be high in AIDS patients with fever and malaise, and the diagnosis made from smears and culture of appropriate samples.

Treatment and outcome

Myco. avium-intracellulare is quite resistant to the usual anti-mycobacterial drugs. It is known to be a difficult infection to treat even in patients without AIDS (Horsburgh *et al.,* 1986). The response to therapy in AIDS patients has been particularly disappointing. Clofazimine and rifabutin are recommended for treatment because most strains of *Myco. avium-intracellulare* are susceptible to them *in vitro.* Evidence of clinical response has been equivocal or poor. Other drugs used in various combinations for the treatment of *Myco. avium-intracellulare* include amikacin, cycloserine, ethionamide, ethambutol and pyrazinamide, all without consistent benefit (Greene *et al.,* 1982; Wong *et al.,* 1985; Hawkins *et al.,* 1986). Regimens using three to six drugs have been used most extensively, without consistent success. Although quantitative cultures have shown a decrease in colony counts in some treated patients, this has not correlated with clinical improvement (Wong *et al.,* 1985). There are reports that occasional patients with AIDS may respond to therapy directed toward *Myco. avium-intracellulare* (Greene *et al.,* 1982; Wong *et al.,* 1985; Horsburgh & Cohn, 1986). Clinical improvement may be related to the in-vitro susceptibility of *Myco. avium-intracellulare* to multiple drugs (Horsburgh & Cohn, 1986). Because *Myco. avium-intracellulare* is the most common mycobacterium isolated from patients with AIDS, some clinicians use the recommended treatment regimen as empirical therapy when smears for acid-fast bacilli are positive, before confirmation of the identity of the organism is available (Centers for Disease Control Report, 1987*b*; Snider *et al.*, 1987). The combination of ciprofloxacin, imipenem/cilastin, and amikacin was shown to be effective in an animal model (Young *et al.*, 1986). In-vitro susceptibility of *Myco. avium-intracellulare* to investigational drugs suggests that BMY-28142, rifapentine and dihydromycoplanicin-A may hold promise for improved treatment.

The prognosis of patients with *Myco. avium-intracellulare* and AIDS is poor. Most patients die with evidence of continued disease despite therapy. Between 1983 and 1985 the CDC (Centers for Disease Control, USA) distributed rifabutin for the treatment of 564 AIDS patients with disseminated *Myco. avium-intracellulare*; the two year survival rate was less than 10% (Snider *et al.*, 1987). Presently a controlled trial is underway comparing rifabutin and rifampicin with a combination of other drugs. Patients who have *Myco. avium-intracellulare* usually have advanced immune suppression and die from other multiple opportunistic infections.

Tuberculosis

Recent reports have stressed the importance of *Myco. tuberculosis* in persons with HIV infection, particularly among the subgroups who abuse drugs or have lived in Haiti or Africa (Pitchenik *et al.*, 1984; Guarner, del Rio & Slade, 1986; Sunderam *et al.*, 1986 Chaisson *et al.*, 1987; Centers for Disease Control Report, 1987*b*; Centers for Disease Control Report, 1987*c* Handwerger *et al.*, 1987; Snider *et al.*, 1987). Earlier in the AIDS epidemic, tuberculosis was felt to be a rare complication in HIV infected homosexuals in the USA. Later studies have shown the incidence of tuberculosis in iv drug users and Haitian patients with AIDS to be 7–20% and 35–69% respectively (Pitchenik *et al.*, 1984; Sunderam *et al.*, 1986; Chaisson *et al.*, 1987; Centers for Disease Control Report, 1987*c*; Handwerger *et al.*, 1987). Other investigators have suggested that, overall, HIV infected patients develop tuberculosis at a higher rate than the general population (Guarner *et al.*, 1986; Chaisson *et al.*, 1987). The development of tuberculosis among AIDS patients may explain the increase in the incidence of the disease observed in the United States over the past several years (Centers for Disease Control Report, 1987*b, c*; Handwerger *et al.*, 1987).

The presence of tuberculosis often seems to preclude demonstration of another opportunistic infection or malignancy. It is postulated that because *Myco. tuberculosis* is highly pathogenic, it may become clinically manifest earlier in the course of immune dysfunction than other opportunistic infections (Pitchenik *et al.*, 1984).

The general distribution of different forms of tuberculosis in patients with HIV infection is shown in Table IV. The presentation of disease is atypical; 60–70% of patients have extrapulmonary disease and 30% have pulmonary disease alone. In contrast, among all cases of tuberculosis in 1980 only 14·0% had non-pulmonary disease (Sunderam *et al.*, 1986). Among AIDS patients, pulmonary tuberculosis alone and extrapulmonary infection alone occur at about an equal frequency (Pitchenik *et al.*, 1984; Chaisson *et al.*, 1987; Handwerger *et al.*, 1987). The most common sites of disease outside the lungs are lymph nodes, blood, urogenital tract, bone marrow and musculoskeletal system. Other reported involved sites include liver, gastrointestinal tract, pericardium, pleura, choroid and rectum (Pitchenik *et al.*, 1984; Croxatto *et al.*,

1986; Sunderam *et al.*, 1986; Chaisson *et al.*, 1987). A tuberculoma must be considered in the aetiology of CNS mass lesions in HIV-infected individuals (Bishburg *et al.*, 1986).

Diagnosis

The consideration of atypical presentations of tuberculosis is appropriate in patients with AIDS. Mycobacterial smear and culture of sputum, blood, bone marrow, urine, stool, lymph node, liver or other tissues with clinical indications can establish the diagnosis. The absence of granuloma formation or the failure to demonstrate organisms by smear does not exclude the diagnosis of tuberculosis; cultures for mycobacteria also should be obtained (Chaisson *et al.*, 1987; Centers for Disease Control Report, 1987*a*). Classical apical infiltrates or cavities are not the usual findings in the chest X-ray of AIDS patients with pulmonary tuberculosis. Radiographic involvement may be diffuse or focal or show as a pleural effusion. The chest X-ray may fail to distinguish tuberculosis from PCP or other infections; however enlarged mediastinal and hilar lymph nodes are rare in PCP and occur in a significant number of AIDS patients with pulmonary tuberculosis (Sunderam *et al.*, 1986; Chaisson *et al.*, 1987; Centers for Disease Control Report, 1987*b*). A positive tuberculin skin test has been found in 40% of tuberculous patients with HIV infection, but a negative test is common after the development of AIDS (Pitchenik *et al.*, 1984; Chaisson *et al.*, 1987; Centers for Disease Control Report, 1987*c*).

Therapy

AIDS patients with tuberculosis generally respond well to standard anti-tuberculous treatment. Fatality directly attributable to *Myco. tuberculosis* is uncommon (Pitchenik *et al.*, 1984; Sunderam *et al.*, 1986; Chaisson *et al.*, 1987; Centers for Disease Control Report, 1987*c*). Longitudinal studies of the clinical and bacteriological response in a large number of patients are not available and so the optimal duration of therapy is not known. Present recommendations are to treat tuberculosis in HIV infected patients with isonazid 300 mg/day, rifampicin 600 mg/day, and pyrazinamide 20–30 mg/kg/day or ethambutol 25 mg/kg/day. The latter one or two drugs may be stopped after two months of treatment, but other anti-tuberculous therapy should be continued for a minimum of nine months, and/or until cultures of affected sites have been shown to be negative for at least six months. The association of HIV infection increases the likelihood of relapse after therapy is completed (Centers for Disease Control Report, 1987*b*; Snider *et al.*, 1987).

Prophylaxis

There is little objective information concerning efficacy of isoniazid prophylaxis in HIV infected persons with a positive PPD skin test. Since prophylaxis is known to be of benefit in other groups of patients given immunosuppressive drugs, the use of isoniazid prophylactically for one year in patients who are known to have been tuberculin positive is advisable, and perhaps continued with advancing immunodeficiency. The favourable response of active tuberculosis to anti-tuberculous therapy in HIV infected persons supports the premise that isoniazid prophylaxis can prevent the reactivation of tuberculosis (Centers for Disease Control Report, 1987a; Snider et al., 1987).

Monitoring the toxicity of anti-tuberculous drugs in AIDS patients is difficult. Most patients are simultaneously receiving drugs for different opportunistic infections or diseases. Experience indicates that patients with AIDS have an increased rate of adverse drug reactions in general. Among HIV infected patients treated for tuberculosis, 26% in one report had an adverse reaction to one or more of the anti-tuberculous drugs in the regimen (Chaisson et al., 1987).

Patients who develop tuberculosis often have other opportunistic infections that cause death. It has been observed that the survival time after the diagnosis of tuberculosis in HIV infected patients was only 7·2 months, which did not differ significantly from the time of survival after the diagnosis of AIDS (Chaisson et al., 1987). Further studies are required to delineate the importance of tuberculosis in the long term outcome of patients with AIDS, but early recognition and aggressive treatment can reverse the morbidity caused by tuberculosis.

Acknowledgements

We are grateful to Mrs Maureen Measure, Department of Virology, The London Hospital Medical College, for the preparation of the manuscript.

References

Bishburg, E., Sunderam, G, Reichman, L. & Kapila, R. (1986). Central nervous system tuberculosis with the acquired immunodeficiency syndrome and its related complex. *Annals of Internal Medicine* **105**, 210–3.

Brivet, F., Livartowski, J., Herve, P., Rain, B. & Dormant, J. (1987). Pericardial cryptococcal disease in the acquired immunodeficiency. *American Journal of Medicine* **82**, 1273.

Centers for Disease Control Report. (1986). Update, acquired immunodeficiency syndrome— United States. *Morbidity and Mortality Weekly Report* **35**, 17–21.

Centers for Disease Control Report. (1987a). Revision of the CDC surveillance case definition for acquired immunodeficiency syndrome. **36**, *Suppl.* 15.

Centers for Disease Control Report. (1987b). Diagnosis and management of mycobacterial infection and diseases in persons with human immunodeficiency virus infection. *Annals of Internal Medicine* **106**, 254–256.

Centers for Disease Control Report. (1987c). Tuberculosis and acquired immunodeficiency syndrome—New York City. *Morbidity and Mortality Weekly Report* **36**, 785–90, 795.

Chaisson, R., Schecter, G., Theuer, C., Rutherford, G., Echenberg, D. & Hopewell, P. (1987). Tuberculosis in patients with the acquired immunodeficiency syndrome. Clinical features, response to therapy, and survival. *American Review of Respiratory Diseases* **136**, 570–4.

Clotet, B., Grifol, M., Parra, O., Boix, J., Junca, J., Tor, J. et al. (1986). Asymptomatic esophageal candidiasis in the acquired immunodeficiency syndrome-related complex. *Annals of Internal Medicine* **105**, 145.

Croxatto, J., Mestre, C., Puente, S. & Gonzalez, G. (1986). Non-reactive tuberculosis in a patient with acquired immune deficiency syndrome. *American Journal of Ophthalmology* **102**, 659–60.

Damsker, B. & Bottone, E. (1985). *Mycobacterium avium-Mycobacterium intracellulare* from the intestinal tracts of patients with the acquired immunodeficiency syndrome, concepts regarding acquisition and pathogenesis. *Journal of Infectious Diseases* **151**, 179–80.

Dismukes, W. (1988). Cryptococcal meningitis in patients with AIDS. *Journal of Infectious Diseases* **157**, 624–8.

Eng, R., Bishburg, E. & Smith, S. (1986a). Cryptococcal infections in patients with acquired immune deficiency. *American Journal of Medicine* **81,** 19–23.

Eng, R., Bishburg, E., Smith, S., Geller, H. & Kapila, R. (1986b). Bacteremia and fungemia in patients with acquired immune deficiency syndrome. *American Journal of Clinical Pathology* **86,** 105–7.

Enhi, W. F. & Ellison, R. T. (1987). Spontaneous *Candida albicans* meningitis in a patient with the acquired immune deficiency syndrome. *American Journal of Medicine* **83,** 806–7.

Farman, J., Tavitian, A., Rosenthal, L., Schwarz, G. & Raufman, J. P. (1986). Focal esophageal candidiasis in acquired immunodeficiency syndrome. *Gastrointestinal Radiology* **11,** 213–7.

Gal, A., Koss, M., Hawkins, J., Evans, S. & Einstein, H. (1986). The pathology of pulmonary cryptococcal infections in the acquired immunodeficiency syndrome. *Archives of Pathology and Laboratory Medicine* **110,** 502–7.

Gillin, J. S., Urmacher, C. & West, R. (1983). Disseminated *Mycobacterium avium-intracellulare* infection in acquired immunodeficiency syndrome mimicking Whipple's disease. *Gastroenterology* **85,** 1187–91.

Gold, J. (1985). Clinical spectrum of infections in patients with HTLV III associated diseases. *Cancer Research* **45,** *Suppl.,* 6425s–7s.

Greene, J., Sidhu, G., Lewin, S., Levine, J., Masur, H., Simberkoff, M. *et al.* (1982). *Mycobacterium avium-intracellulare,* a cause of disseminated life-threatening infection in homosexuals and drug abusers. *Annals of Internal Medicine* **97,** 539–46.

Guarner, J., del Rio, C. & Slade, B. (1986). Tuberculosis as a manifestation of the acquired immunodeficiency syndrome. *Journal of the American Medical Association* **256,** 3092.

Handwerger, A., Mildvan D., Senie, R. & McKinley, F. W. (1987). Tuberculosis and the acquired immunodeficiency syndrome at a New York City Hospital 1978–1985. *Chest* **91,** 176–80.

Hawkins, C., Gold, J., Whimbey, E., Kiehn, T., Brannon, P., Cammarata, R. *et al.* (1986). *Mycobacterium avium* complex infections in patients with the acquired immunodeficiency syndrome. *Annals of Internal Medicine* **105,** 184–8.

Heinemann, M., Bloom, A. & Horowitz, J. (1987). *Candida albicans* endophthalmitis in a patient with AIDS. *Archives of Ophthalmology* **105,** 1172–3.

Holmberg, K. & Meyer, R. (1986). Fungal infections in patients with AIDS and AIDS-related complex. *Scandinavian Journal of Infectious Diseases* **18,** 179–92.

Horsburgh, C. & Cohn, D. L. (1986). *Mycobacterium avium* complex and the acquired immunodeficiency syndrome. *Annals of Internal Medicine* **105,** 969.

Horsburgh, C., Cohn, D., Roberts, R., Masur, H., Miller, R., Tsang, A. & Iseman, M. (1986). *Mycobacterium avium—M. intracellulare* isolates from patients with or without acquired immunodeficiency syndrome. *Antimicrobial Agents and Chemotherapy* **30,** 955–7.

Kiehn, T., Edwards, F., Brannon, P., Tsang, A., Maio, M., Gold, J. *et al.* (1985). Infections caused by *Mycobacterium avium* complex in immunocompromised patients, diagnosis by blood culture and fecal examination, antimicrobial susceptibility tests, and morphological and seroagglutination characteristics. *Journal of Clinical Microbiology* **21,** 168–73.

Kiehn, T. & Cammarata, R. (1986). Laboratory diagnosis of mycobacterial infections in patients with acquired immunodeficiency syndrome. *Journal of Clinical Microbiology* **24,** 708–11.

Klein, R. S., Harris, C., Small, C. B., Moll, B., Lesser, M. & Friedland, G. H. (1984). Oral candidiasis in high risk patients as the initial manifestation of acquired immune deficiency. *New England Journal of Medicine* **311,** 354–7.

Kovacs, J., Kovacs, A., Polis, M., Craig Wright, W., Gill, V. J., Tuazon, C. *et al.* (1985). Cryptococcosis in the acquired immune deficiency syndrome. *Annals of Internal Medicine* **103,** 533–8.

LaFont, A., Wolff, M., Marche, C., Clair, B. & Regnier, B. (1987). Overwhelming myocarditis due to *Cryptococcus neoformans* in an AIDS patient. *Lancet ii,* 1145–6.

Levine, M. S., Woldenberg, R., Herlinger, H. & Laufer, I. (1987). Opportunistic esophagitis in AIDS, radiographic diagnosis. *Radiology* **165,** 815–20.

Levy, R., Bredesen, D. & Rosenblum, M. (1985). Neurologic manifestations of the acquired immunodeficiency syndrome (AIDS), experience at UCSF and review of the literature. *Journal of Neurosurgery* **62,** 475–95.

Lief, M. & Sarfarazi, F. (1986). Prostatic *Cryptococcus* in acquired immune deficiency syndrome. *Urology* **28,** 318–9.

Macher, A., Kovacs, J., Gill, V., Roberts, G., Ames, J., Park, C. *et al.* (1983). Bacteremia due to *Mycobacterium avium-intracellulare* in the acquired immunodeficiency syndrome. *Annals of Internal Medicine* **99**, 782–5.

Masur, H., Tuazon, C., Gill, V., Grimes, G., Baird, B., Fauci, A. *et al.* (1987). Effect of combined clofazimine and ansamycin on *Mycobacterium avium-Mycobacterium intracellulare* bacteremia in patients with AIDS. *Journal of Infectious Diseases* **155**, 127–9.

Perla, E., Maayan, S., Miller, S., Ramaswamy, G. & Eisenberg, H. (1985). Disseminated cryptococcosis presenting as the adult respiratory distress syndrome. *New York State Journal of Medicine* **85**, 704–6.

Pitchenik, A., Cole, C., Russell, B., Fischl, M., Spira, T. & Snider, D. (1984). Tuberculosis, atypical mycobacteriosis, and the acquired immunodeficiency syndrome among Haitian and non-Haitian patients in South Florida. *Annals of Internal Medicine* **101**, 641–5.

Poropatich, C., Labriola, A. & Tuazon, C. (1987). Acid-fast smear and culture of respiratory secretions, bone marrow, and stools as predictors of disseminated *Mycobacterium avium* complex infection. *Journal of Clinical Microbiology* **25**, 929–30.

Reichert, C., O'Leary, T. J., Levens, D. L., Simrell, C. R. & Macher, A. M. (1983). Autopsy pathology in the acquired immunodeficiency syndrome. *American Journal of Pathology* **112**, 357–82.

Rhoads, J., Wright, D., Redfield, R. R. & Burke, D. S. (1987). Chronic vaginal candidiasis in women with human immunodeficiency virus infection. *Journal of the American Medical Association* **257**, 3105–7.

Ricciardi, D., Sepkowitz, D. Berkowitz, L., Bienenstock, H. & Maslow, M. (1986). Cryptococcal arthritis in a patient with acquired immune deficiency syndrome. *Journal of Rheumatology* **13**, 455–8.

Robinson, P., Sulita, M., Matthews, E. & Warren, J. (1987). Failure of the BACTEC 460 radiometer to detect Cryptococcus neoformans fungemia in an AIDS patient. *American Journal of Clinical Pathology* **87**, 783–6.

Roux, P., Touboul, J. L., Feuilhade de Chauvin, M., Delacour, T., Revuz, J., Basset, D. *et al.* (1986). Disseminated cryptococcosis diagnosed in AIDS patients by screening for soluble serum antigens. *Lancet i*, 1154.

Snider, D., Hopewell, P., Mills, J. & Reichman, L. (1987). Position Paper, American Thoracic Society. Mycobacterioses and the acquired immunodeficiency. *American Reviews of Respiratory Diseases* **136**, 492–6.

Stover, D., White, D., Romano, P., Gellene, R. & Robeson, W. (1985). Spectrum of pulmonary diseases associated with the acquired immunodeficiency syndrome. *American Journal of Medicine* **78**, 429–37.

Sunderam, G., McDonald, R., Maniatis, T., Oleske, J., Kapila, R. & Reichman, L. (1986). Tuberculosis as a manifestation of the acquired immunodeficiency syndrome (AIDS). *Journal of the American Medical Association* **256**, 362–6.

Tavitian, A., Raufman, J. P. & Rosenthal, L. (1986a). Oral candidiasis as a marker for esophageal candidiasis in the acquired immunodeficiency syndrome. *Annals of Internal Medicine* **104**, 54–5.

Tavitian, A., Raufman, J. P., Rosenthal, L. E., Weber, J., Webber, C. & Dincsoy, H. (1986b). Ketoconazole-resistant *Candida* esophagitis in patients with acquired immunodeficiency syndrome. *Gastroenterology* **90**, 443–5.

The Medical Letter. (1988). **30**, Issue 761.

Welch, K., Finkbeiner, W., Alpers, C., Blumenfeld, W., Davis, R. L., Smuckler, E. A. *et al.* (1984). Autopsy findings in the acquired immune deficiency syndrome. *Journal of the American Medical Association* **252**, 1152–9.

Whimbey, E., Gold, J., Polsky, B., Dryjanski, J., Hawkins, C., Blevins, A. *et al.* (1986). Bacteremia and fungemia in patients with acquired immunodeficiency syndrome. *Annals of Internal Medicine* **104**, 511–4.

Witt, D., McKay, D., Schwam, L., Goldstein, D. & Gold, J. (1987). Acquired immune deficiency syndrome presenting as bone marrow and mediastinal cryptococcosis. *American Journal of Medicine* **82**, 149–50.

Wolinsky, E. (1979). Nontuberculosis *Mycobacterium* and associated diseases. *American Review of Respiratory Disease* **119**, 107–59.

Wong, B., Edwards, F., Kiehn, T., Whimbey, E., Donnelly, H., Bernard, E. *et al.* (1985).

Continuous high-grade *Mycobacterium avium-intracellulare* bacteremia in patients with the acquired immune deficiency syndrome. *American Journal of Medicine* **78**, 35–40.

Young, L., Inderlied, C., Berlin, O. G. & Gottlieb, M. (1986). Mycobacterial infections in AIDS patients, with an emphasis on the *Mycobacterium avium* complex. *Reviews of Infectious Diseases* **8**, 1024–33.

Zakowski, P., Fligie, S., Berlin, G. & Johnson, L. (1982). Disseminated *Mycobacterium avium-intracellulare* infection in homosexual men dying of acquired immunodeficiency. *Journal of the American Medical Association* **248**, 2980–2.

Zuger, A., Louie, E., Holzman, M., Simberkoff, M. & Rahal, J. (1986). Cryptococcal disease in patients with the acquired immunodeficiency syndrome. *Annals of Internal Medicine* **104**, 234–40.

Journal of Antimicrobial Chemotherapy (1989) **23**, *Suppl. A*, 127–135

Diagnosis and treatment of Kaposi's sarcoma

Margaret F. Spittle

*The Meyerstein Institute of Radiotherapy and Oncology,
The Middlesex Hospital, Mortimer Street, London W1N 8AA, UK*

Kaposi's sarcoma occurs in the non-classical form in immunosuppressed patients in non-HIV patients in Africa and in patients infected with HIV. The latter group are now the most common. The treatment of Kaposi's sarcoma in AIDS patients must be seen in the context of their general condition. Symptomatic treatment by radiotherapy and low dose chemotherapy is often all that is appropriate. Immunotherapy has a small treatment role at present.

Introduction

Non-epidemic Kaposi's sarcoma is a rare disease. Until five years ago the most commonly seen variant in this country was the classical variety described by Kaposi in 1972 (Kaposi, 1982). This occurs in the elderly European Jewish population and patients from the Mediterranean area, with a ten to one preponderance of men.

In general, the disease initially affects the lower legs, appearing as small raised, dark red or violet nodular lesions, almost always associated with ankle oedema. The lesions may be few or many and form indurated plaques or protruding nodules which may break down and bleed. The disease is multifocal and although one foot may be affected before the other, eventually both are usually the site of multiple Kaposi lesions which increase in size, become more numerous and spread in a centripetal direction (Figure 1). There is often early involvement of the penis and hands. Lesions can affect the whole of the skin, the upper airways, gastrointestinal tract, lungs and lymph nodes. However, in general it is an extremely slowly progressive disease and in many patients, no treatment is necessary at all as symptoms are minimal. Kaposi's sarcoma is relatively radiosensitive and local radiotherapy to the local and regional areas affected can be given (Cohen, 1982). Chemotherapy also produces a moderately good response.

Kaposi's sarcoma also occurs in immunosuppressed individuals—those having azothiaprine to prevent rejection of renal transplants are probably the biggest group. Men and women are equally affected. The disease may regress following cessation of the immunosuppressive therapy (Solan, Greenwald & Silvay, 1981).

Kaposi's sarcoma unrelated to HIV infection or immunosuppression has always been found in subSaharan East-Central Africa. This disease affects a younger age group and is more rapidly progressive than that seen in Europe and America. Massive exophytic tumours may be seen especially of the lower limbs (Figure 2). There is a lymphadenopathic variety which affects children. Chemotherapy has been used widely and with some success in the treatment of African Kaposi's sarcoma as radiotherapy

127

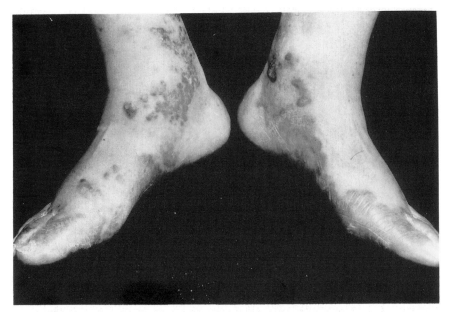

Figure 1. (a) Kaposi's sarcoma of feet and lower legs in an elderly Jewish man.

has not been available in the centres where this variant of Kaposi's sarcoma is seen (Olweny, Toya & Katongole-Mbidde, 1974). However the local response to moderate doses of radiotherapy is dramatic.

Epidemic Kaposi's sarcoma

The most common form of Kaposi's sarcoma now seen in clinical practice in Great Britain is that associated with HIV infection. Up to 40% of homosexual patients with AIDS have Kaposi's sarcoma and a diagnosis of Kaposi's sarcoma in an HIV positive person is diagnostic of AIDS (Figure 3). However, less than 10% of intravenous drug abusers and haemophiliacs exhibit Kaposi's sarcoma as part of their HIV infection. The African AIDS patients also have a very low incidence of Kaposi's sarcoma and HIV infection accounts for less than 10% of African patients with Kaposi's sarcoma. It is not known why this disease should be so prominent in the homosexual community. It has been suggested that exposure to a virus may be a co-factor and cytomegalovirus has been particularly cited. There has been a reduction in the incidence of Kaposi's sarcoma in AIDS patients in San Francisco from 1981–1985. This fall parallels that of a fall in the rate of CMV seroconversion in observed seronegative homosexual men over the same time period (Drew & Huang Eng-shang, 1988).

In the homosexual community Kaposi's sarcoma often presents as a prodrome of opportunist infections, and since patients become diagnosed as having AIDS because of the occurrence of Kaposi's sarcoma, often a considerable time elapses before an opportunist infection (Volberding, 1988) supervenes. The homosexuals with Kaposi's sarcoma therefore are always among the AIDS patients with the best prognosis. Why the Kaposi's sarcoma lesions should appear during this prodromal phase is unknown. When, however, Kaposi's sarcoma is first seen after the patient has developed his first opportunist infection, the prognosis is the same as for other AIDS patients with

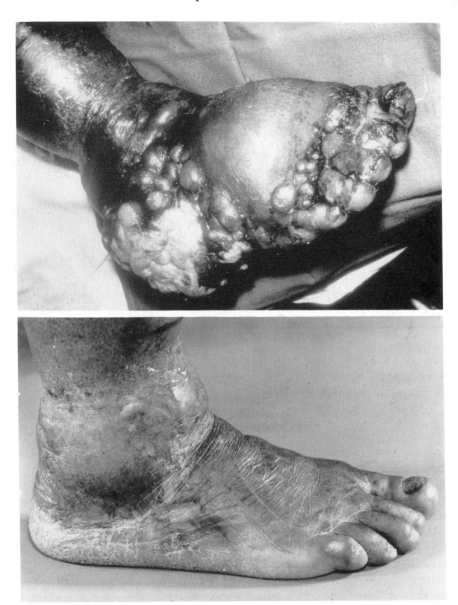

Figure 2. Kaposi's sarcoma of foot of patient from Africa, before (top), and seven years after local radiotherapy (bottom).

opportunist infections. Kaposi's sarcoma itself is rarely the cause of death in a patient with AIDS.

Pathology

Kaposi's sarcoma is a malignant multifocal lesion which either arises from, or is related to, the vascular endothelium of lymphatics or blood vessels. Considerable controversy has arisen over the histogenesis of Kaposi's sarcoma and is discussed by Dorfman (Dorfman, 1984).

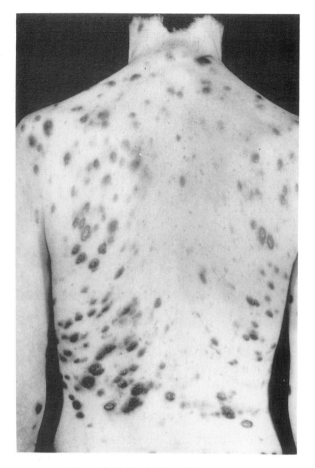

Figure 3. Epidemic Kaposi's sarcoma.

The histopathological interpretation of lesions of Kaposi's sarcoma becomes increasingly difficult when small samples of tissue from organs other than skin, i.e. needle biopsy of lungs and lymph nodes, are obtained. The early skin lesions show irregular, long spaces in the dermis with surrounding haemosiderin and chronic inflammatory cells. The lymphangiomatous type of Kaposi's sarcoma shows anastomosing spaces with very little evidence of tumour cells. The nodular variety shows grouping of spindle cells in the dermis, trapping red cells, and with associated haemosiderin (Figure 4).

Clinical diagnosis

The clinical diagnosis of Kaposi's sarcoma of the skin is not normally difficult and rarely warrants a biopsy to confirm it. The lesions are multiple at an early stage and their colour characteristic. Unlike the lesions in the elderly Jew the lower legs are not usually the most affected site. Multiple plaque-like and nodular patches occur, particularly on the trunk, face and limbs. Often the older lesions become darkly stained and infiltrated, but are not always the largest. Involvement of the palate is frequent causing bleeding and instability of teeth. The upper airways and the rectum

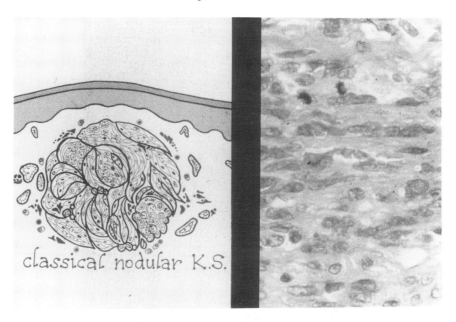

Figure 4. Pathology of Kaposi's sarcoma.

are also commonly affected. Kaposi's sarcoma of the lung is one of the causes of breathlessness, cough and haemoptysis in patients with AIDS.

Treatment

The treatment of Kaposi's sarcoma must be seen in the context of the HIV infection from which the patient is suffering. In general, the treatment policy is dictated by the general condition of the patient. Symptoms of Kaposi's sarcoma can readily be divided into non-life threatening and life threatening.

The most common problem arising with non-life threatening Kaposi's sarcoma is cosmetic. Red lesions on the face and arms are easily seen and can be disfiguring and isolating (Figure 5). Local radiotherapy is easily given and is not generally immunosuppressive. One or two fractions of radiation of superficial voltage is sufficient to stop the treated lesion increasing in size, to cause regression and to decrease pigmentation.

Lesions around the feet which may bleed respond well, drying up after a short course of radiotherapy (Figure 6). This makes the management of these patients on the wards and at home easier. The precise radiotherapy regimen for these localized cosmetic lesions is variable. One dose of 800 cGy at 100 kV is sufficient to control a specific lesion for three to six months. If the patients prognosis is good, a higher dose can be given by increasing the number of fractions of treatment or the single dose may be repeated later (Spittle, 1987) (Figure 7).

Involvement of the palate is a particularly common and distressing feature of Kaposi's sarcoma and the soggy gums which result may bleed and cause instability of the teeth. 400 cGy given on five occasions by opposing supervoltage fields across the palate gives good lasting regression of the disease (Smith & Spittle, 1987).

A small, but definite number of patients seem to have an idiosyncratic reaction to

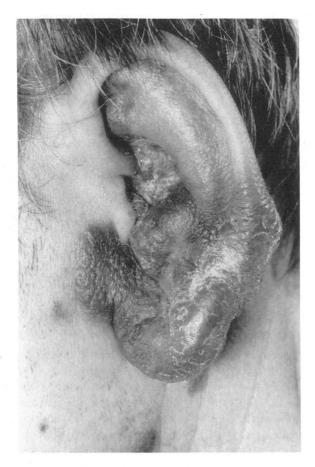

Figure 5. Kaposi's sarcoma of the ear.

radiation on mucosal surfaces and get an alarming mucositis. This does not seem to be due to concurrent infection with candida nor to be obviously drug related. This aggressive mucositis may be due to proximity of radiotherapy with immunosuppressive or cytotoxic treatment, but has not been explained. Increased fractionation with lower doses per fraction is appropriate when irradiating the mucosal surfaces. Widespread gross facial oedema is another distressing complication of Kaposi's sarcoma in AIDS and irradiation to the whole face with supervoltage treatment giving 2000 cGy in two weeks is often sufficient to control this distressing symptom. Involvement of the upper airways may be life threatening, with nodules of Kaposi's sarcoma sometimes causing complete laryngeal obstruction. Radiotherapy—3000 cGy in three weeks with supervoltage treatment—can cause complete regression. Treatment with radiotherapy is thus effective and lasting in the management of Kaposi's sarcoma.

Widespread Kaposi's sarcoma, which may be painful and extremely cosmetically distressing, can also be treated with chemotherapy and immunotherapy. In a patient who has not had any opportunist infections and in whom the prognosis is relatively good, full chemotherapy may be given. Regimens including etoposide, vincristine and bleomycin have been recorded as giving a 40 to 60% response rate (Lewis, Abrams & Ziegler, 1983). There is no evidence that the use of multiple agents is more effective

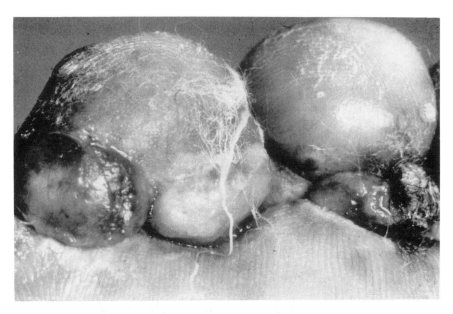

Figure 6. Kaposi's sarcoma of the toes—note bleeding.

than single agent chemotherapy. Immunotherapy with interferon has the potential advantage of not precipitating immunosuppression and therefore has been used in patients after their first opportunist infection (Groopman, Gottlieb & Goodman, 1984). The high doses—30–50 mega-units given subcutaneously daily or every second day—needed to control the Kaposi's sarcoma may have considerable side-effects. A flu-like illness, fever, nausea, shivering and headaches are commonly seen and may be extremely distressing, causing discontinuation of therapy. The patient with Kaposi's sarcoma who has already had the first opportunist infection related to HIV disease must be treated carefully. Cytotoxic agents are best reserved for life threatening disease, as these patients have a poor tolerance of chemotherapy. Unfortunately, chemotherapy tends to precipitate the opportunist infections from which these patients most frequently die.

A particularly distressing life threatening complication of Kaposi's sarcoma is involvement of the lung. Nodular involvement of the mediastinum or lymphangitic spread through both lung fields and pleural effusions are frequently seen. The dyspnoea associated with the disease may be improved with whole lung irradiation, giving 150 cGy on 13 occasions to a total dose of 1950 cGy by opposing fields with supervoltage. Nodular disease in the mediastinum may be treated by local radiotherapy with supervoltage which gives good symptomatic control. Gross involvement of the bowel or massive intra-abdominal lymphadenopathy may also respond to moderate doses of radiotherapy. Immunotherapy as described above can also be used. A five day infusion of low-dose bleomycin with the addition of vincristine is well tolerated and can be repeated every three weeks as long as the white blood count remains above 3000 mm^3. Although the response rate is about 50%, some patients do get a good lasting remission from this treatment. Although side-effects with this regimen are minimal and bone marrow toxicity *per se* is rarely seen, in AIDS patients haemoglobin, WBC and platelets frequently fall due both to the infection and to the

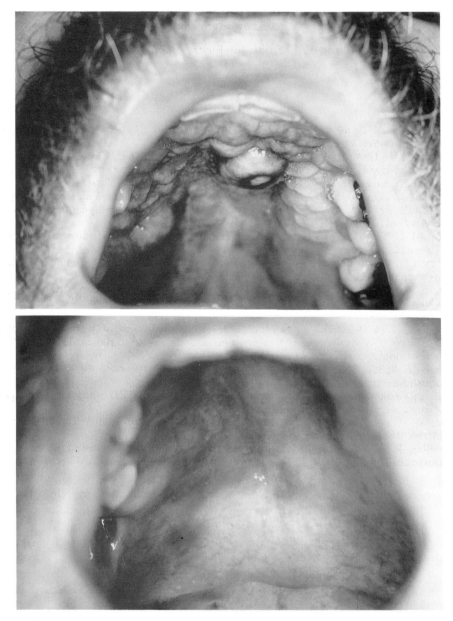

Figure 7. Kaposi's sarcoma of the palate, before (top) and after (bottom) radiotherapy.

drugs used to treat them (notably zidovudine). Leiderman studied bone-marrow regenerating capacity in 18 AIDS patients and suggested that a factor inhibitory to myelopoiesis is present (Leiderman *et al.*, 1984).

In general therefore the management of AIDS patients with Kaposi's sarcoma must be considered in the context of their general disease state. Radiotherapy has a prominent part to play and, although chemotherapy can be successful, it may precipitate the opportunist infections to which patients may succumb. Immunotherapy has a poorer response rate and can give considerable toxicity.

Acknowledgements

I should like to thank Dr N. P. Smith for Figure 4 and Miss Elizabeth Pratt for her encouragement and secretarial assistance.

References

Cohen, L. (1962). Dose, time and volume parameters in irradiation therapy and Kaposi's sarcoma. *British Journal of Radiology* **35,** 484–8.

Dorfman, R. F. (1984). Kaposi's sarcoma revisited. *Human Pathology* **15,** 1013–7.

Drew, W. L. & Huang Eng-shang (1988). Role of cytomegalovirus. In *Kaposi's Sarcoma* (Ziegler, J. L. & Dorfman, R. F., Eds), pp. 113–28. Marcel Dekker, New York.

Groopman, J., Gottlieb, M. & Goodman, J. (1984) Recombinant alpha-2 interferon therapy of Kaposi's sarcoma associated with acquired immune deficiency syndroma. *Annals of International Medicine* **100,** 671–6.

Kaposi, M. (1982). Classics in oncology. Idiopathic multiple pigmented sarcoma of the skin. *Cancer* **32,** 342–7.

Leiderman, I. Z., Greenberg, M. L., Adelsberg, B. R. & Siegal, F. P. (1984). Defective myelopoiesis in AIDS. *Journal of Cell Biochemistry, Suppl. 8A, 14.*

Lewis, B., Abrams, D. & Ziegler, J. (1983) Single agent or combination chemotherapy of Kaposi's sarcoma in acquired immune deficiency syndrome. *American Society of Clinical Oncology* **2,** 59.

Olweny, C., Toya, T. & Katongole-Mbidde, E. (1974). Treatment of Kaposi's sarcoma by combination of actinomycin-D, vincristine and imidazole carboximide (NSC-45388). *International Journal of Cancer* **14,** 649–56.

Smith, N. & Spittle, M. F. (1987). Tumours. *ABC of AIDS* (Adler, M. W., Ed.). pp. 19–22. British Medical Journal, London.

Solan, A., Greenwald, E. & Silvay, O. (1981). Long-term complete remissions of Kaposi's sarcoma with vinblastine therapy. *Cancer* **47,** 637–9.

Spittle, M. F. (1987). A simple and effective treatment for AIDS related Kaposi's sarcoma. *British Medical Journal* **295,** 248–9.

Volberding, P. A. (1988). Clinical features and staging. In *Kaposi's Sarcoma* (Ziegler, J. L. & Dorfman, R. F., Eds), pp. 169–87. Marcel Dekker, New York.

Index